Medical Imaging - Principles and Applications

Edited by Yongxia Zhou

Published in London, United Kingdom

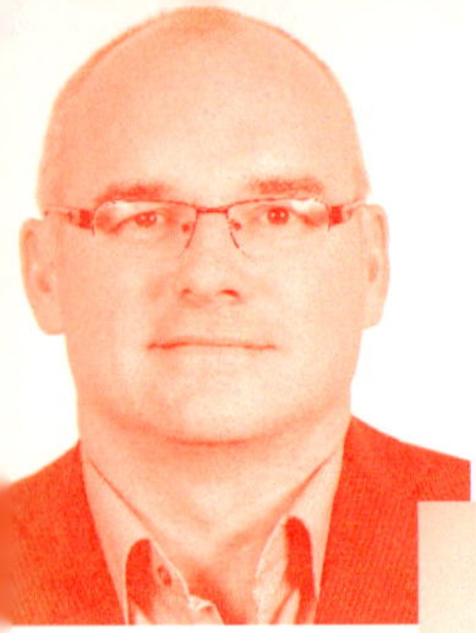
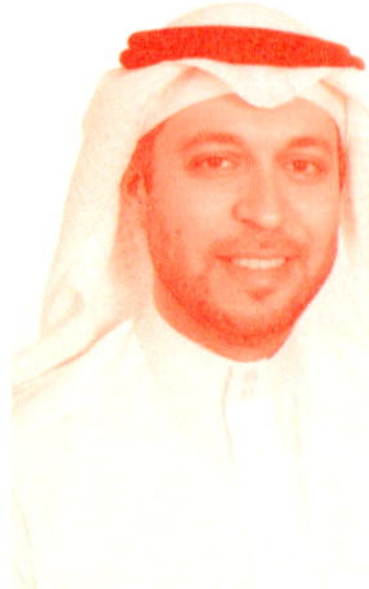
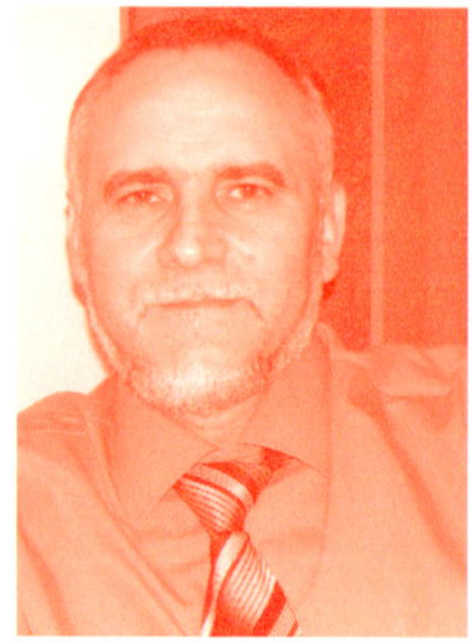
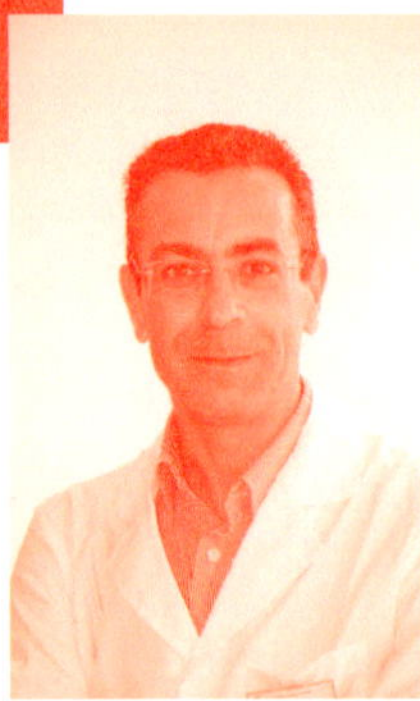
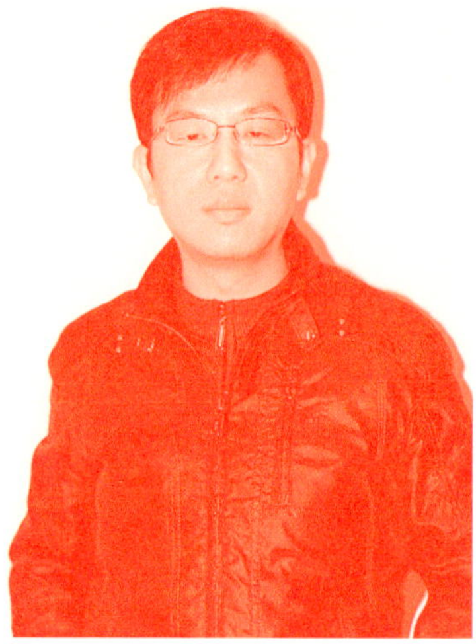
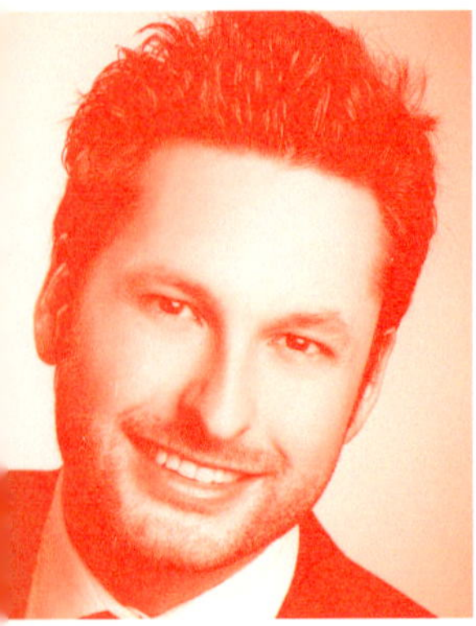
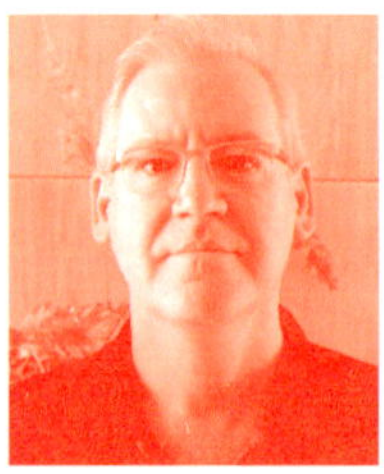

IntechOpen

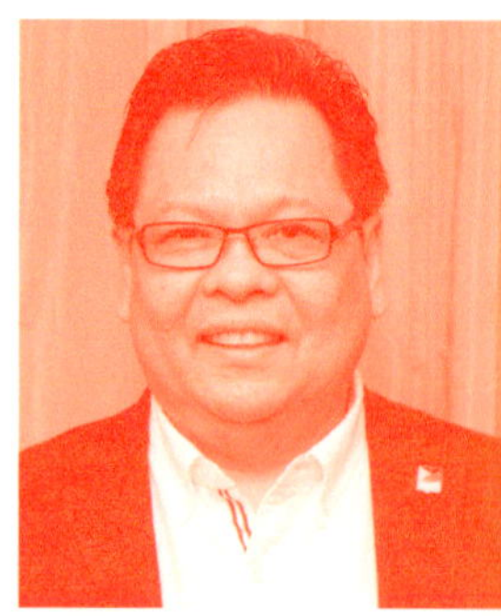
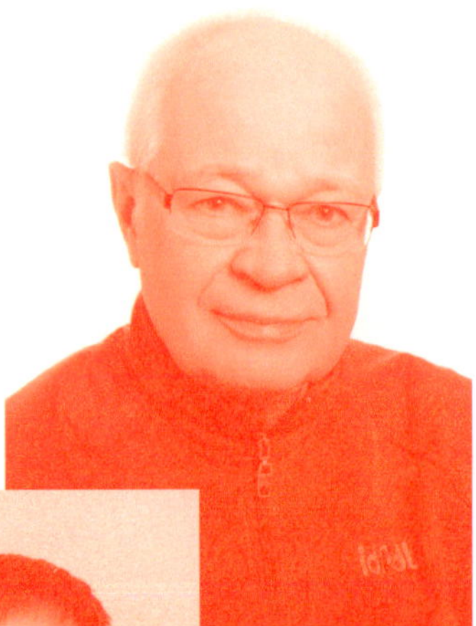
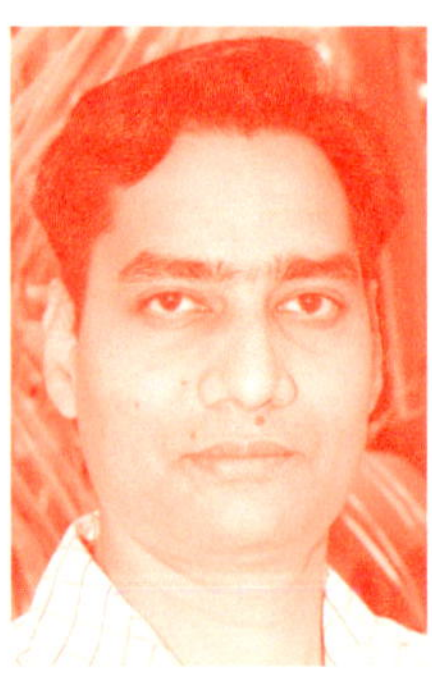
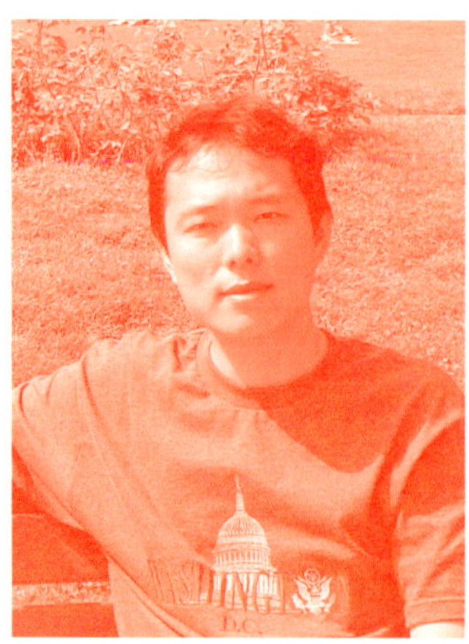
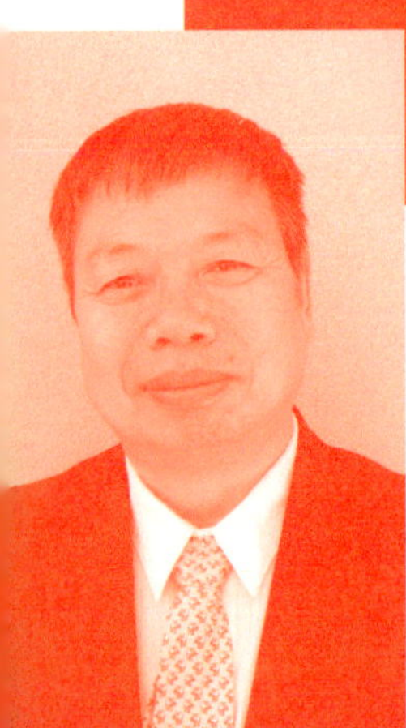
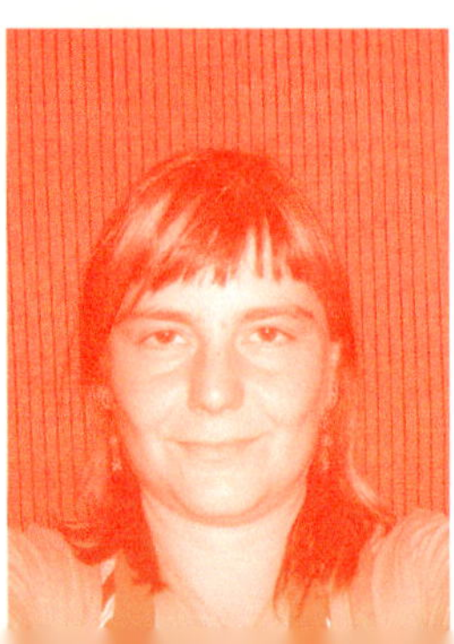

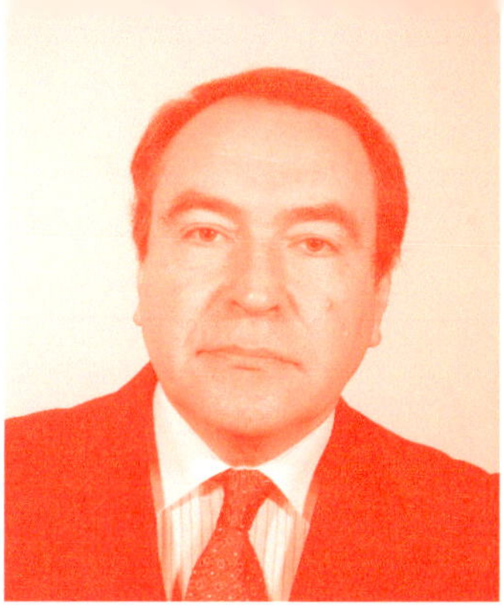

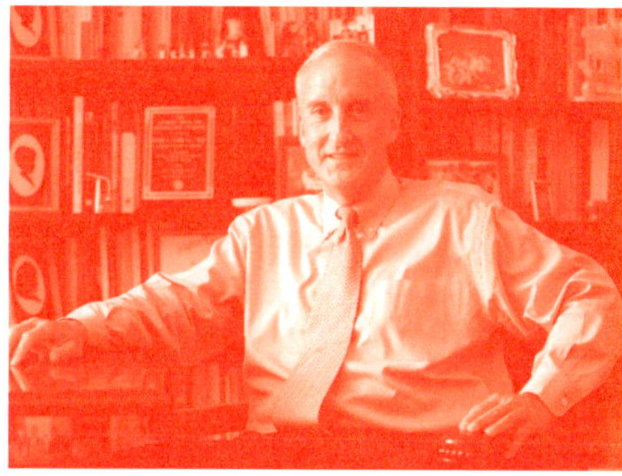

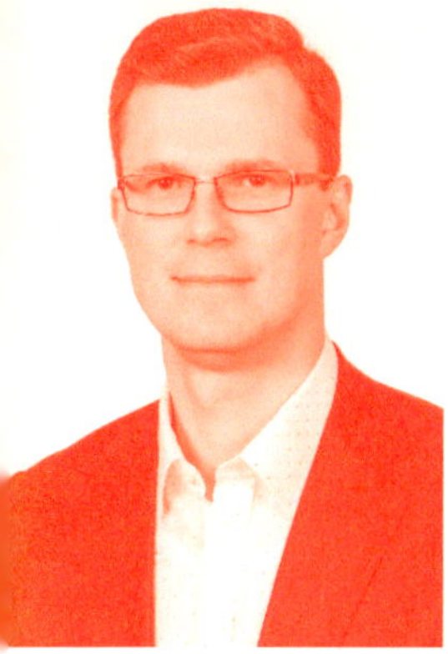

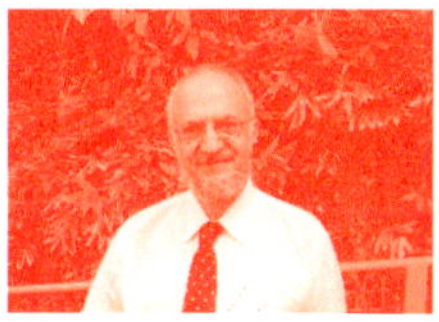

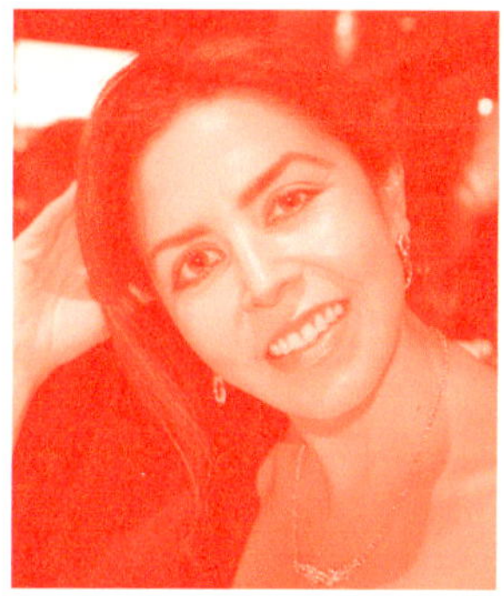

Supporting open minds since 2005

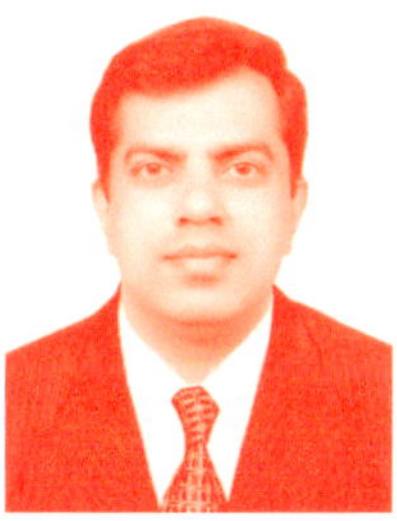

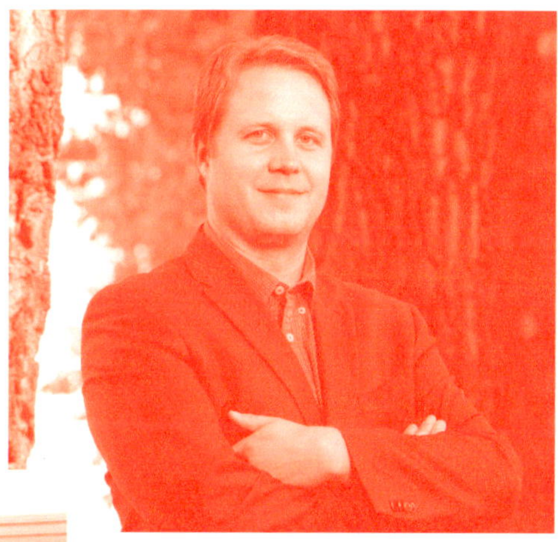

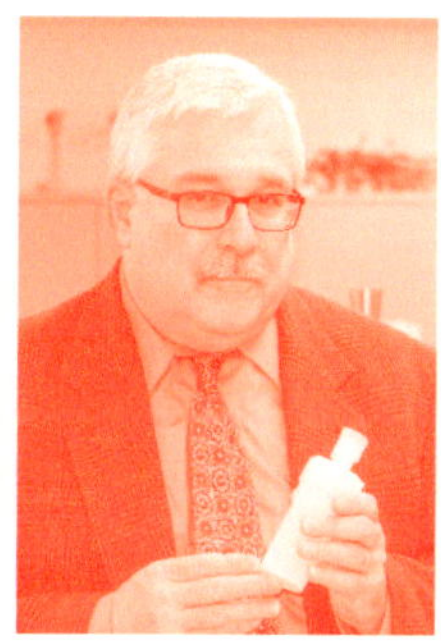

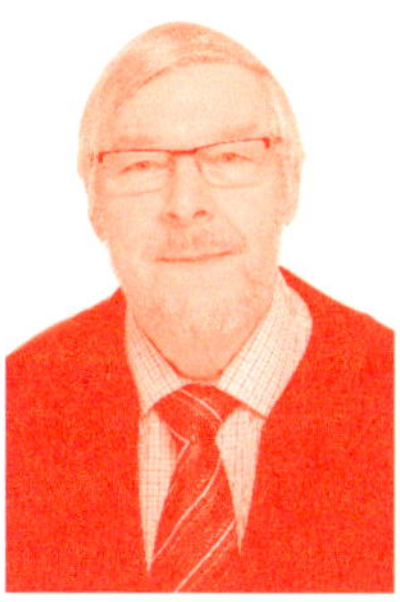

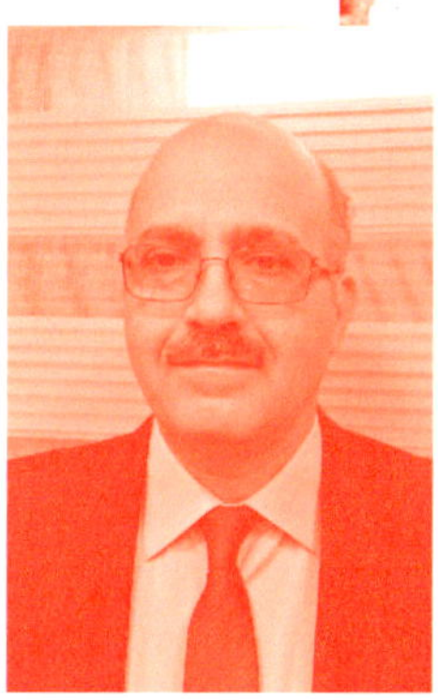

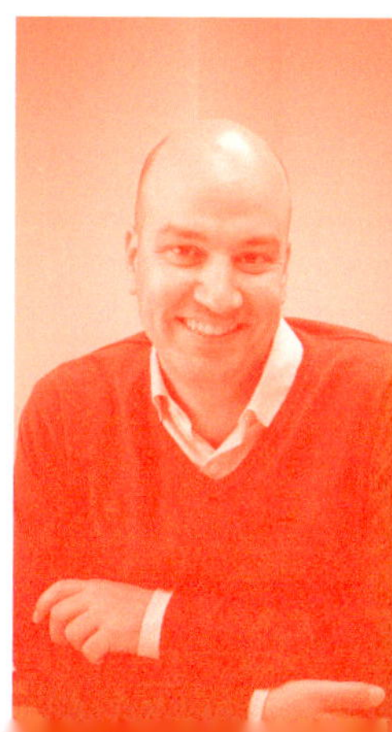

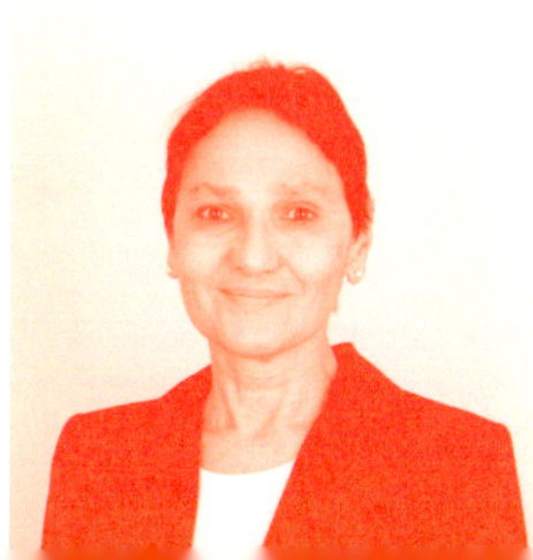

Medical Imaging - Principles and Applications
http://dx.doi.org/10.5772/intechopen.78073
Edited by Yongxia Zhou

Contributors
Yongxia Zhou, Yousif Mohamed Y. Abdallah, Tariq Alqahtani, Long Chen, Yunchao Huang, Hua Sun, Evangelos Gazis, Zhi Dou, Liqiang Yang

First published in London, United Kingdom, 2019 by IntechOpen
IntechOpen is the global imprint of INTECHOPEN LIMITED, registered in England and Wales, registration number: 11086078, 7th floor, 10 Lower Thames Street, London, EC3R 6AF, United Kingdom
Printed in Croatia

British Library Cataloguing-in-Publication Data
A catalogue record for this book is available from the British Library

Additional hard and PDF copies can be obtained from orders@intechopen.com

Medical Imaging - Principles and Applications
Edited by Yongxia Zhou
p. cm.
Print ISBN 978-1-78923-871-6
Online ISBN 978-1-78923-872-3
eBook (PDF) ISBN 978-1-78985-724-5

For EU product safety concerns:
IN TECH d. o. o., Prolaz Marije Krucifikse Kozulić 3, 51000 Rijeka, Croatia, info@intechopen.com or visit our website at intechopen.com.

Meet the editor

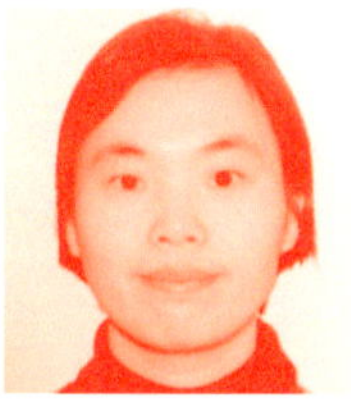

Yongxia Zhou completed her PhD from the University of Southern California in Biomedical Imaging in 2004. Her research interest is radiology and neuroscience applications. She was trained and worked as a neuroimaging scientist in several prestigious institutes, including Columbia University, University of Pennsylvania, and NIH. Her research focuses on multimodal neuroimaging integration, including MRI/PET and EEG instrumentation and makes best use of multiple modalities to help interpret underlying disease mechanisms. She has authored more than five monograph books, and edited several books for well-known publishers, including IntechOpen and Nova Science. She has published more than 100 papers and abstracts in and served as reviewer and editor for many reputable international journals and conferences.

Contents

Preface

Medical imaging is a rapidly growing field with recent tremendous technical developments. Great achievements have been made regarding disease diagnosis from basic science to clinical applications. Most well-known imaging modalities include the widely used magnetic resonance imaging (MRI), positron-emission tomography (PET), and X-ray computed tomography (CT). With the high-resolution imaging acquisitions and advanced imaging processing methods, accurate and precise functional, structural, and molecular images can be applied to patients to improve diagnosis and treatment. Several distinct imaging perspectives such as cutting-edge imaging methods from principles to data analysis, better correlation with neurocognitive function, as well as detailed examples and summaries of disease monitoring could help convey the methodological, technical, and developmental information of medical imaging principles and applications.

The first section of the book provides functional MRI (fMRI) and structural imaging techniques and applications. Chapter 1 assesses baseline and longitudinal functional and structural connectivity changes associated with age and gender at both baseline and longitudinal follow-up time points. Correlation with neurocognitive data from a large sample of healthy older adults and apolipoprotein E (APOE) genotypic effects has been investigated thoroughly. The strengths of this study are the extensive and well-characterized large sample of older adults and multiple imaging metrics, including advanced fMRI, multiple structural imaging to capture extensive properties of functional connectivity, activity, and white matter integrity, and myelination. The results in this chapter are presented with full-spectrum quantification of neuroimaging and neurocognitive/genetopic data with significant impact on the longitudinal neuroimaging application field. Chapter 2 describes the brain regions of neuropathic pain studied with fMRI techniques, including resting state and task fMRI and structural changes. The introduction of fMRI techniques and central mechanisms of neuropathic pain, including pain perception and processing in the brain, stages of pain (chronic), and two types of pain (hyperalgesia vs. allodynia), are covered in detail. The significance of fMRI in the treatment of neuropathic pain has been evaluated, including consistent quantification of pain intensity, treatment efficacy, and non-invasive transcranial stimulation application. This review chapter provided readers with the current status and future directions of fMRI technology to better serve the clinic and assist in the diagnosis and prognosis of neuropathic pain.

The second section of the book covers the imaging principles of X-ray radiation, PET, and applications in cancer. Chapter 3 gives a detailed and quantitative description of radiation interaction, substance absorption, and PET/CT imaging detection systems. The principles of ionizing radiation interaction with matter and participant are introduced for different particles, including photons, electrons, and heavy charged particles. Different types of possible attenuations and absorptions are covered. Radiation detectors and data acquisition as well as reconstruction systems of several imaging modalities are described. The strong points of this chapter are accurate formula layout and illustrative figures. Chapter 4 investigates PET/CT (with anatomy details from CT and metabolism information from PET) applications in lung cancer diagnosing, staging, and treatment. Several aspects, including clinical features, classification, grading, and pathology of lung cancer, principles of PET/CT, and evaluation of diagnosing and treatment, are reviewed. This chapter gives a good example of cancer imaging diagnosis and applications, including detailed demonstrations of each cancer sub-type, staging criteria, and classification, as well as better clinical evaluations.

The third section refers to the imaging processing technique and its development. Chapter 5 gives an overview of the medical imaging processing perspectives from principles to post-analysis applications. Medical imaging is developing rapidly due to developments in imaging processing techniques, including image recognition, analysis, and enhancement. Several imaging modalities used for disease diagnosis and processing methods, including registration, segmentation, and edge detection, are described as well. This chapter presents multiple examples of image analysis application, and illustrates commonly used image processing algorithms for higher spatial and temporal resolution as well as better clinical interpretation.

Yongxia Zhou, PhD
University of Southern California and Columbia University,
Los Angeles, California, USA

Section 1

Magnetic Resonance Imaging and Applications

Chapter 1

Longitudinal Changes of Structural and Functional Connectivity and Correlations with Neurocognitive Metrics

Yongxia Zhou

Abstract

Revealing brain functional and micro-structural changes over a relatively short period at individual levels are especially important given that many risks associated with age including vascular and neuroinflammation increases and could confound the baseline fMRI parametric images. Cellular-level axonal injury and/or demyelination as well as dispersed mesoscopic level substance abnormal aggregation and structural/functional abnormality could occur in short subacute/acute phases, while literatures related to longitudinal changes with age are limited with only our previous fMRI findings. Longitudinal data were used to characterize these multiparameters including random intercept and interval per individual. No significant age by gender interactions have been found to either DTI fractional anisotropy (FA) or diffusivity metrics. The interval effective regions showed longitudinal change of FA and radial diffusivity (RD)/axial diffusivity (AX) values remained similar to the aging results found with cross-sectional data. Significant correlations between DTI and fMRI metrics as well as between imaging and neurocognitive data including speed and memory were found. Our results indicate significant and consistent age, gender and apolipoprotein E (APOE) genotypic effects on structural and functional connectivity at both short-interval and cross-sectional ranges, together with correlational neurocognitive functions.

Keywords: microstructure, function connectivity, DTI, longitudinal change, neurocognitive test, correlation, age, APOE gene

1. Introduction

Functional connectivity based on MRI (fcMRI) measures simultaneous and synchronous neuronal activities at various regions connected intrinsically in brain with functional MRI time courses. In our recent study, we reported lower functional connectivity in posterior cingulate and temporal regions with aging within the default mode network (DMN) [1]. We also found higher fcMRI in the dorso-attentional network (DAN) (including in the dorso-lateral prefrontal cortex) at age, which could be due to the negative connectivity with DMN. Furthermore longitudinal changes in fcMRI occurred in regions similar to those demonstrating cross-sectional effects of age, with only a few small brain areas showing significant age by interval or gender by interval effects. The rate of fcMRI longitudinal change, however, was not influenced significantly by baseline age or gender, after adjusting for baseline age and gender modulation effects in majority of brain regions, suggesting moderate linear interval effects of fcMRI longitudinal changes in brain. Our results from this relatively large cohort suggest that fcMRI variability from various networks in different scales might be useful to monitor brain changes in normal aging and preclinical stages of Alzheimer's disease [1]. As for diffusion tensor imaging (DTI), we used both voxel-wise four DTI metrics and tract-specific ROI analysis to investigate myelin and axonal integrity differences with age, gender and APOE genotype with four DTI metrics at baseline [2–5]. One of the main findings was the decreased fractional anisotropy (FA) but increased radial diffusivity (RD) with age based on both voxel-wise and tract-specific analyses indicating both axonal degeneration and demyelination [6, 7]. Dramatic decreases of FA with age, especially in participants over 50 years old, accompanied by increased RD suggest that white matter (WM) integrity declines with age. In contrast, changes in axial diffusivity (AX) and mean diffusivity (MD) with age are in two-way: higher AX and MD in some tracts and cortical regions including bilateral thalamic radiation and cingulum bundles, as well as decreased AX and MD in some long-distance fasciculus [8–11].

Regarding DTI and fMRI correlations, significant gray matter (GM) and WM correspondences based on GM atrophy and WM fractional anisotropy (FA) reductions in several brain regions were found in multiple sclerosis (MS) patients including primary visual cortex/optic radiation as well as somatosensory cortex/superior longitudinal fasciculus at baseline [12]. However, with disease progresses, these associations might be deteriorated and are not maintained [13–15], although each imaging feature at baseline and longitudinal time points remain consistent and highly correlated [16, 17]. The degree of change (or rate of change) of each metric is dependent on the sensitivity during the disease course [18–20]. For instance, GM atrophy and functional coordination decrement were found at follow-up visit in MS patients, in contrast to the usual observation of significant FA reductions and WM lesions predominantly in corpus callosum, periventricular areas, occipital horns and cingulum areas at baseline in MS compared to controls [12]. In mild traumatic brain injury (MTBI), 1 year after injury, there was measurable global brain atrophy, larger than that in control subjects. The anterior cingulate WM bilaterally and the left cingulate gyrus isthmus WM, as well as the right precuneal GM, showed significant decreases in regional volume in patients with MTBI over the 1st year after injury [21]. However at baseline, after normalization to supratentorial brain volume, there were no significant regional brain volume differences between patients with MTBI at the time of their initial visit and the control group. Our observations complement these findings and indicate that specific brain structure such as the cingulum and precuneus may be more vulnerable to long-term structural changes [22, 23].

It had been reported that baseline imaging findings including micro-structure integrity measured with DTI can predict functional activation and coordination at follow-ups. We had reported that FA measure at baseline predicted follow-up functional coordination score from fMRI data ($r = 0.68$, $P = 0.007$), indicating a possible initial WM inflammatory factor to the subsequent neurodegenerative processes in MS patients [12]. We also found that baseline composite imaging metrics can predict cognitive function and neuropsychological scores. For instance, in MTBI, the clinical symptom at follow-up visit could be predicted with high accuracy from baseline imaging features with $r = -0.82$, $P < 0.001$ for depression; $r = -0.65$, $P = 0.01$ for anxiety; $r = -0.71$, $P = 0.005$ for fatigue; and $r = -0.67$, $P = 0.008$ for post-concussion syndrome (PCS) [23]. Revealing the brain micro-structural changes over a relatively short period at individual levels are especially important given that many risks associated with age including vascular and neuroinflammation increases and could confound the baseline parametric images of each individual. However, literatures related to longitudinal changes of neuroimaging data with age are still limited [24].

The goals of this study were to assess baseline and longitudinal age and gender-related changes with neuroimaging and neurocognitive data from a large sample of healthy older adults, as well as apolipoprotein E (APOE) genotypic effects. The strengths of this study are the extensive and well-characterized large sample of older adults, and multiple imaging metrics including advanced fcMRI, four DTI (FA, MD, RD, AX) to capture extensive properties of functional connectivity and white matter myelination at both baseline and longitudinal follow-up time points. Both conventional whole brain voxel-wise analyses and fiber track-specific ROI quantification measures that are more robust and less prone to registration error were used to increase the white matter myelin detection specificity. Beside previous fcMRI findings [1], we also investigate longitudinal changes of multiple DTI and fMRI metrics as well as neurocognitive tests. The correlations among different imaging metrics as well as between neuroimaging findings and neurocognitive scores were quantified to better illustrate the full spectrum of multiple phenotypic data.

2. Methods

2.1 Participants

We studied 572 cognitively normal participants in the neuroimaging substudy from the Baltimore Longitudinal Study of Aging (BLSA) who had DTI assessments. Exclusion criteria were as follows: subjects with excessive motions and unwanted imaging qualities (N = 17 and 30 scans); subjects with incidental findings of brain lesions or other central nervous diseases, such as, Parkinson's disease (N = 4). Twenty individuals aged 24–39, 39 individuals aged 40–49, 51 aged 50–59, 137 aged 60–69, 186 aged 70–79, and 138 aged 80–89.

Three hundred and eighty-seven participants (68%) had available APOE genotype information, 107 APOE ε4+ and 280 APOE ε4− participants were further divided into six sub-groups based on the APOE isoforms. These sample characteristics are shown in **Table 1**. Two hundred and forty-five subjects had longitudinal follow-up (interval range 0.9–3.5 years, mean interval of 1.9 ± 0.6 years) and were used to characterize aging effects at short interval. Neurocognitive data from 21 cognitive tests with 59 variables that measure multiple cognitive functionalities including visual perception and attention, learning and memory encoding and recall, language fluency, and executive function for each participant was collected at the same day of the MRI scan [25]. After post-processing with normalization, 52 test scores were used for further analysis including correlation tests.

2.2 Imaging parameters

MRI imaging was obtained with a 3T whole-body scanner (Philips, Achieva) at National Institute of Aging, using an eight-channel head coil. The DTI sequence was evaluated previously and found to have good intra-site reliability and inter-section reproducibility [1]. Specifically, standard echo-planar imaging (EPI)-based DTI protocol was performed during the routine 45-min scan (TR/TE = 6801/75 msec, flip angle = 90°, FOV = 212 × 212 mm^2, spatial resolution = 0.83 × 0.83 × 2.2 mm^3, 65 slices to cover the whole cerebrum). Thirty-two diffusion gradient directions (diffusion gradient time Δ = 36.3 ms and pulse duration δ = 16 ms) with b-factor of 700 s/mm^2 and a total of 3:58 min for each run as well as two identical runs were obtained for each subject.

Characteristic	All DTI baseline	ε4/ε4	ε3/ε4	ε2/ε4	ε3/ε3	ε2/ε3	ε2/ε2	Both DTI and fMRI
Total n	572	4	95	8	219	59	2	236
Age, years; mean ± SD	69.7 ± 13.4	68.4 ± 16.8	67.0 ± 12.1	69.4 ± 12.6	70.1 ± 11.3	70.0 ± 10.1	75.9 ± 16.4	72.0 ± 12.2
Gender n; women/men	311/261	3/1	56/39	7/1	115/104	30/29	1/1	135/101
Education, years; mean ± SD	17.1 ± 2.7	17.5 ± 1.0	17.4 ± 2.5	17.1 ± 2.1	16.9 ± 2.6	17.6 ± 2.2	16.0 ± 2.8	17.0 ± 2.4
MMSE at visit	28.6 ± 1.5	28.3 ± 1.5	28.8 ± 1.4	29.5 ± 0.6	28.4 ± 1.6	28.5 ± 1.4	29.0 ± 1.4	28.8 ± 1.3

Table 1.
Sample characteristics for the whole sample and six APOE genotypic sub-groups.

A standard echo-planar imaging (EPI) resting-state (RS)-fMRI protocol (TR/TE = 2000/30 msec, flip angle = 75°, FOV = 240 × 240 mm^2, voxel size =3 × 3 × 4 mm^3, 37 slices) was performed during an approximately 45-min brain MRI protocol. A total of 180 volumes were acquired during the 6-min RS-fMRI scan. Participants were instructed to remain still, with eyes open and focused on a cross fixation, and encouraged to relax during the scan. A 3-dimensional T1-weighted MPRAGE (magnetization prepared rapid gradient-echo imaging) sequence (TR/TE/TI = 6.8/3.2/849.2 msec, FA = 8°, FOV = 192 × 256 × 256 mm^3, voxel size = 1.2 × 1 × 1 mm^3) was acquired in sagittal-view for segmentation of tissue types and registration/normalization of EPI images to MNI space.

2.3 Image processing

DTI data were first pre-processed with the diffusion toolkit toolbox (http://trackvis.org) to obtain the FA/RD/AX/RD values in original b0 space. For the FA/RA/AX/RD quantification, the FMRIB, Software Library (FSL, http://fsl.fmrib.ox.ac.uk/fsl) tract-based spatial statistics toolbox steps 1–2 (i.e., preprocessing, brain mask extraction with FA > 0.2 and normalization) were used for registration of all participants' FA into the FSL 1-mm white matter skeleton template. The transformation of the individual FA data to the FSL Montreal Neurological Institute (MNI) template with 1-mm isotropic voxel size, was implemented with the nonlinear registration tool FNIRT based on a b-spline representation of the registration warp field. After normalization of FA map to the MNI space, tract-specific mean FA values were obtained in 20 regions from the well-defined probabilistic tract template (FSL/JHU ICBM atlas). Quantitative MD/AX/RD values were obtained by applying the same transformation from individual FA to template space and computed with tract-specific values [1].

The anatomic T1-MPRAGE and 4D EPI functional data were preprocessed using both FSL and Analysis of Functional NeuroImages (AFNI) programs (adapted scripts from http://www.nitrc.org/projects/fcon_1000 developed based on FSL and AFNI). For structural MPRAGE data used for fMRI data normalization, preprocessing included reorientation to the right-posterior-inferior convention and skull stripping, and segmentation into three tissue types: GM, WM, and cerebrospinal fluid (CSF). The segmental tissue masks were used to derive the nuisance fMRI signals in WM and CSF. Finally, the MPRAGE image was co-registered with the fMRI data and normalized to the Montreal Neurologic Institute (MNI) 152-brain template with 2-mm isotropic voxel size [1, 12].

For fcMRI processing, the first four volumes of the RS-fMRI data of each subject were discarded for scanner and image stability. Preprocessing steps for RS-fMRI data included rigid alignment of the time frames using AFNI motion correction algorithms, spatial smoothing using a Gaussian kernel with 6 mm full-width-at-half-maximum (FWHM), and band-pass temporal filtering of 0.005–0.1 Hz to improve signal-to-noise ratio. Removal of nuisance signals was then performed using a Gaussian regression model after co-registration to MPRAGE data. Namely, motion parameters, global signal, and signals derived from CSF and WM based on the tissue masks were modeled in the Gaussian linear mixed model, and residual signal at each voxel was maintained for further analyses. Finally the residual 4D fMRI data after regression were transformed to MNI standard space [26]. A DMN seed including both medial prefrontal cortex (MED) (MNI center: 0, 48, 23 mm) and posterior cingulate cortex (PCC) (MNI center: 26, 248, 39 mm) with a combined volume of 4112 mm^3 (each seed of 2056 mm^3) was used. We refer to this seed as the combined core seed. We chose the combined core seed over separate PCC and MED seeds because the latter approach generates different and incomplete DMN connectivity patterns [27], whereas the combined core seed yields consistent and complete depictions of DMN [26]. Whole brain voxel-wise Pearson correlation coefficients were computed between the average time series within the seed and the time course of each fMRI voxel in the brain. Finally Z-statistics were derived voxel-wise. 2nd-level Gaussian random field (GRF) and family-wise corrections were applied to derive the functional connectivity (FC) map with FSL toolbox.

In addition to the combined core seed, the fcMRI generated from other seeds were also evaluated to study the systematic-level fcMRI, with a total of 26 seeds [1]. The other 25 seeds included 12 conventional regions of different sub-areas of DMN (e.g., PCC and intra-parietal sulcus), three thalamic (left, right, and whole thalamus) and seven subthalamic seeds [28], and three subcortical seeds (caudate and putamen from the MNI template, and hypothalamus from an in-house developed probability map) [29]. The conventional 12 seeds were derived from the script seed library (http://www.nitrc.org/projects/fcon_1000), including the hippocampal formation and frontal eye field (FEF) seeds that generated the task-positive networks (i.e., these networks are more active at task-conditions, in contrast to resting state). All seeds were well-evaluated and validated previously [27, 28, 30]. The global mean Z-values were obtained from the fcMRI maps generated from each of 26 seeds to study age and gender effects as well, by averaging the fcMRI Z-maps over the whole brain with a threshold of GRF cluster-corrected $P < 0.01$.

Meanwhile in the resting state, fractional amplitude of low-frequency fluctuations (fALFF) has been shown to be higher in the DMN regions that are active and it had also been reported that task-related (e.g., working memory, motor visual stimuli and cognitive tasks) alterations of low-frequency oscillations could reflect real-time neuronal activity [28]. The idea of fALFF method was to scale the summary of amplitude at low-frequency band (e.g., 0.01–0.08 Hz) to the summary of amplitude across whole band to remove white and physiological noise. In this study, the resting-state fALFF Z-value at baseline and longitudinal changes of fALFF, as well as correlations with the age and other fcMRI/DTI neuroimaging metrics were performed from 236 participants with available data resource.

2.4 Statistical analyses

For DTI, effects of age, gender and APOE genotype were studied at both whole-brain voxel-wise level and tract-specific ROI analyses using the four DTI metrics-FA, RD, AX and MD. Linear mixed effects (LME) model was applied to characterize both baseline and longitudinal effects of age, gender and age by gender interactions of the four metrics [1, 31]. We used the MATLAB Statistics toolbox (www.mathworks.com, R2015b) and in-house programs to perform model fitting as listed in Eq. (1). Longitudinal data were incorporated to characterize the longitudinal change of DTI metrics with interval as the prediction parameter as well. In order to account for within-individual correlations stemming from follow-up data, we included random intercept and random interval (i.e., random slope) terms per individual in LME.

$$\begin{aligned} \text{DTI} \sim & \beta_0 + \beta_1 \text{ gender} + \beta_2 \text{ baseage} + \beta_3 \text{ interval} \\ & + \beta_4 \text{ interval:baseage} + \beta_5 \text{ gender:baseage} + \beta_6 \text{ interval:gender} \end{aligned} \tag{1}$$

For whole-brain analyses, voxel-wise linear regression with DTI metrics as the dependent variable and age as an independent variable using SPM12 software (Statistical Parametric Mapping, http://fil.ion.ucl.ac.uk/spm/software/spm12) was implemented. Gender term was included as a covariate. Then two-sample t-test comparison using baseline DTI data was also implemented to study gender differences between women and men, and age was used as a covariate [32].

For tract-specific ROI-based analyses, the mean value of each regional FA and diffusivity (i.e., RD, AX and MD) analysis were quantified with FSL toolbox and in-house programs developed with MATLAB (www.mathematics.com). Both linear and quadratic fitting were used to examine white matter myelination along aging trajectories. Mean values of all six APOE genotypes were derived from each ROI to form the waveform and multiple-group comparisons of the four DTI metrics stratified by genotypic isoforms were performed in MATLAB toolbox.

To characterize cross-sectional and longitudinal changes in fcMRI, we used a LME model, similar to DTI longitudinal data model with the same analyses algorithm as listed in Eq. (2). In order to account for cross-sectional differences across individuals, we included baseline age and gender as covariates. Baseline age was centered at group mean of 69.4 years. Men were coded as 0.5 and women as −0.5. Time interval in years between baseline and follow-up was included to capture longitudinal change in fcMRI. We also included interaction terms with interval, random intercept and interval terms to compute longitudinal rates of fcMRI change accounting for baseline age and gender interactions [1].

$$\text{fcMRI} \sim \beta 0 + \beta 1\ \text{baseage} + \beta 2\ \text{gender} + \beta 3\ \text{interval} + \beta 4\ \text{interval:baseage} + \beta 5\ \text{gender:baseage} + \beta 6\ \text{interval:gender} \quad (2)$$

Conventional statistical comparison (with relatively smaller number of participants) using a two-sample t-test at baseline and 3 years follow-ups, adjusting for gender, with the same statistical threshold as used in LME model ($P < 0.01$ and cluster size ≥10 voxels) was used for longitudinal fALFF data quantification. To validate the age and gender effects observed in LME model, SPM-based conventional regression model including general linear correlational analysis between age and fcMRI adjusted for gender, and comparison between women and men group adjusted for age were performed as well.

3. Results

3.1 Age effects on DTI

Whole brain DTI FA showed prominent aging effects (i.e., reduced FA with aging) in the main projections fibers including cingulum bundle and superior longitudinal fasciculus ($P < 0.00001$) (**Figure 1a**). The monotonically reduction of FA was observed in relatively older subject with age larger than 50 years old that construe the majority of the sample size. RD, on the other hand, showed only significantly higher RD values with age in bilateral thalamic radiations, bilateral somatosensory cortex, visual cortex, anterior and posterior cingulate gyri, middle temporal cortex including hippocampus, subcallosal cortex and posterior cerebellum ($P < 0.01$, cluster size = 10). Very small clusters and primarily in the cerebellum was found to have lower RD along the age (**Figure 1b**). Axial diffusivity showed significantly higher AX values with age in some similar regions to RD including bilateral thalamic radiations, bilateral somatosensory cortex, visual cortex, posterior cerebellum and superior corona radiata tract ($P < 0.01$, cluster size = 10). In contrast to RD and FA, AX was also significantly lower in white matter regions including bilateral cortico-spinal tract, inferior longitudinal fasciculus, optic radiation and cerebellum (**Figure 1c**). MD shows almost a similar aging pattern as of AX (**Figure 1d**) [1].

As expected, all the tract-based ROI showed significant aging effects (i.e., reduced FA with age) after adjustment for multiple comparisons ($r = 0.3$–0.7, mean $r = 0.5$, corrected $P < 0.0001$). Quadratic fitting of FA from 20 track-specific ROIs showed

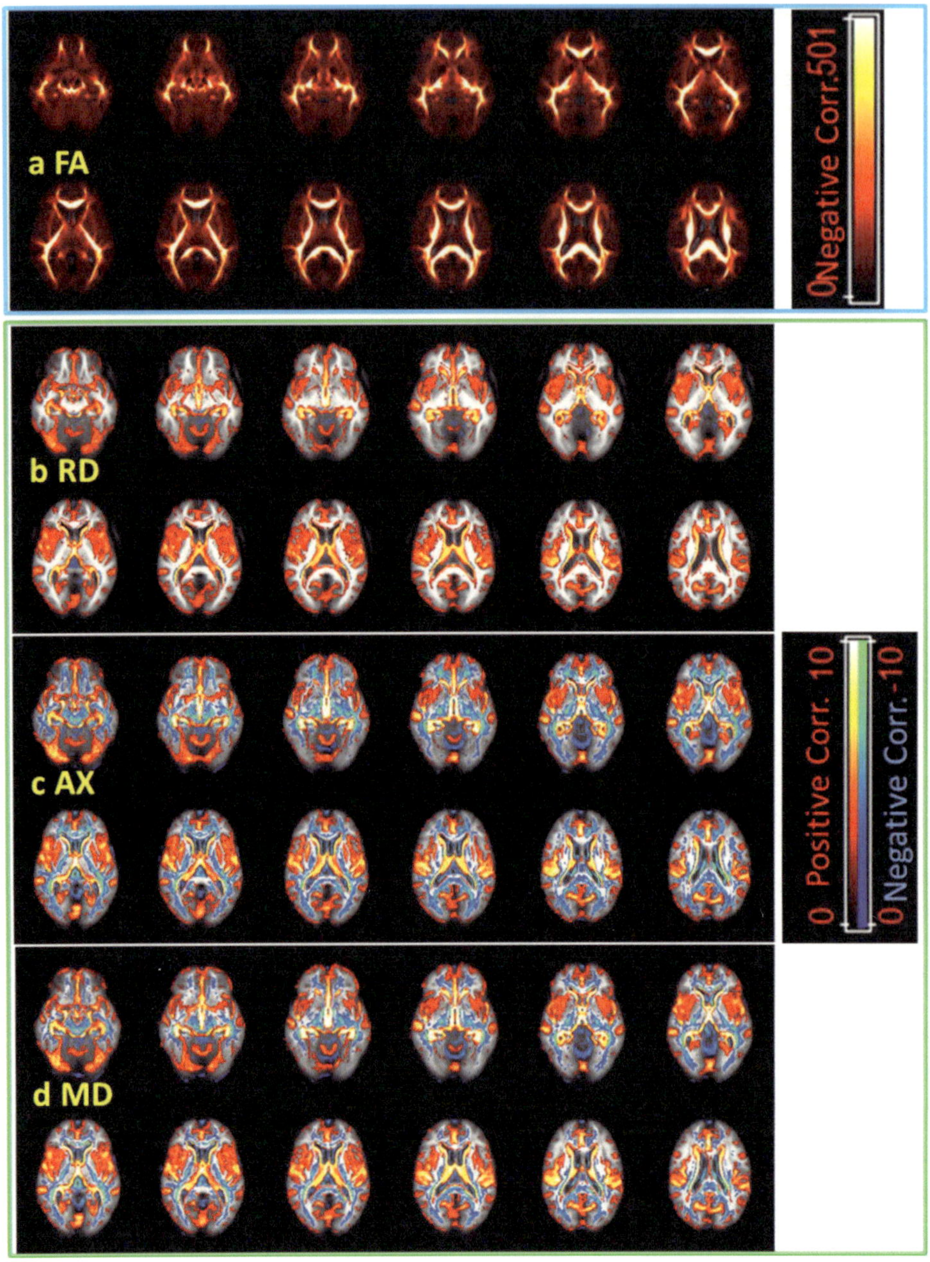

Figure 1.
(a) Prominent aging effects were demonstrated with negative correlation between voxel-wise FA and age, i.e., decreased FA along the age (statistical T map, P < 0.01, cluster size = 10) for all brain regions. On the other hand, RD was increased along the age for some of the brain regions including somatosensory cortex and cingulum bundle (b). There are both increases and decreases of AX (c) and MD (d) in different brain regions along the age, and the changes of AX and MD have very similar patterns (all P < 0.01, cluster size = 10). Background image was derived from average of all subjects' FA maps in MNI space.

aging trajectories with maturation age (i.e., mean FA reaches maximum) falling between [24, 28–41] years. The relatively earlier maturation age was found in the major forceps and bilateral thalamic radiation (28–33 years) and later maturation age from bilateral hippocampal portion of the cingulum and corticospinal tracts (39–42 years) (**Figure 2**). The tract-based ROI that has the earliest maturation age with highest FA at 27.9 years is the major forceps. The left hippocampal portion of the cingulum bundle

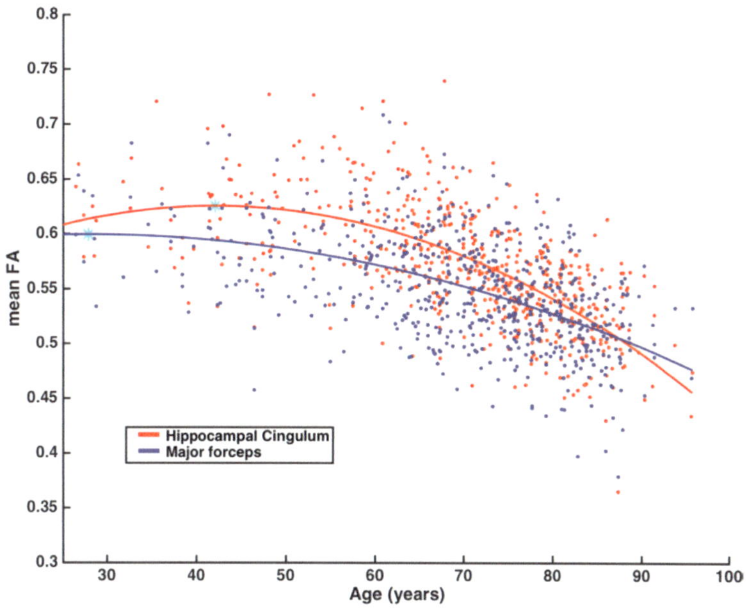

Figure 2.
Quadratic aging trajectories of two tract-specific ROIs. Star (cyan color) indicates maturation age when mean FA of the tract each tract-specific ROI reaches maximum. Major forceps has the earliest maturation age, with highest FA at 27.9 years (blue color). While the left hippocampal portion of the cingulum bundle has the latest maturation age, with highest FA at 42.1 years (red color).

has the latest maturation age (42.1 years). While the diffusivity measures from tract-based ROIs showed mostly linearly increases of diffusivity along the age with RD, and some tracts showed no significant aging effects based on AX or MD [1].

Using diffusion toolkit (http://www.nitre.org/projects/trackvis/) with an advanced tensorline propagation algorithm for fiber tracking, we found tracts that play important roles in memory and cognitive function also illustrated significant aging effects, including fiber tract numbers of the fornix that connects the hippocampus to the whole brain, and fibro bundles connecting bilateral parahippocampus to the whole brain were decreased significantly with aging (both $P < 0.00001$).

3.2 Longitudinal change of FA

Based on LME model, no significant age by gender interactions have been found to either FA or diffusivity metrics in the whole-brain voxel-wise analyses indicating aging and gender effects can be studied independently (**Figure 3a**). The interval effective regions estimated from LME model showed longitudinal change of FA and RD/AX values remained similar to the aging results found with cross-sectional data as in **Figure 1** and gender effective brain regions ($P < 0.01$, cluster size = 10) (**Figure 3b**).

3.3 Gender effects on DTI

We found men had significantly higher FA in the hippocampal portion of the cingulum bundle, secondary somatosensory cortex, thalamus, cingulate and cerebellar regions compared to women, based on voxel-wise FA comparisons ($P < 0.01$). Lower FA in men than women in bilateral inferior longitudinal fasciculus, anterior thalamic radiation, frontal cortex and temporal part of the superior longitudinal fasciculus were also observed ($P < 0.01$, cluster size = 10). Scattered cortical regions including superior frontal, cerebellum and insular showed higher RD in men than women, and lower RD

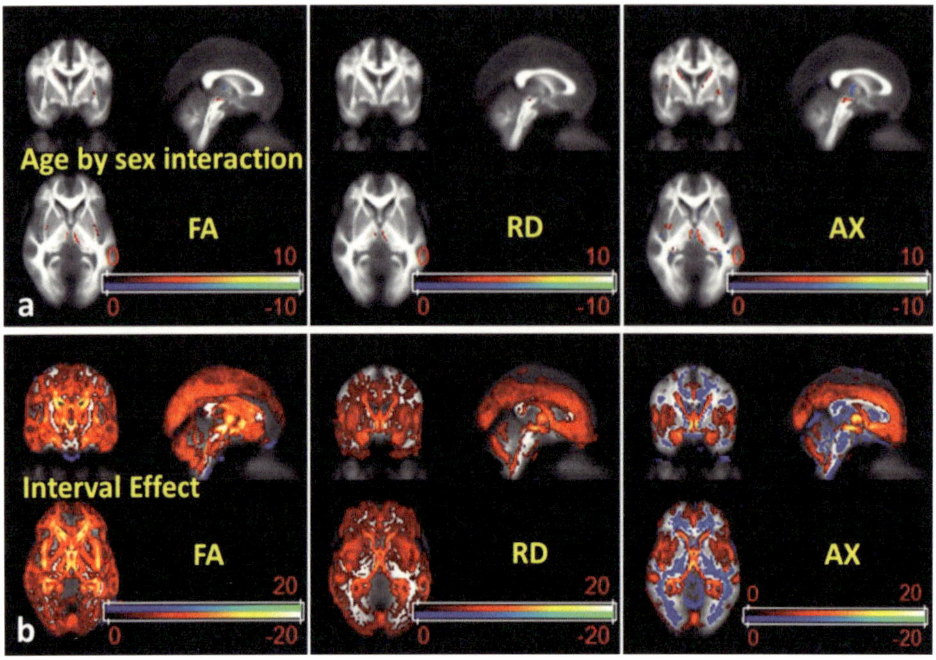

Figure 3.
(a) Based on LME model, no significant age by gender interaction of DTI FA and diffusivity values across whole-brain with only a few outliers (P < 0.01). (b) The interval effect estimated from LME model using longitudinal data showed longitudinal change of FA, RD and AX values (MD is almost the same as AX) in brain regions similar to the baseline aging effects (1–3 years of interval of follow-up time; P < 0.01, cluster size = 10), suggesting an observable longitudinal change within a short time interval.

in men only with small clusters in cerebellum. Furthermore AX and MD values in most of brain regions were higher in men than women (P < 0.01, cluster size = 10).

3.4 APOE genotype effects

Voxel-wise FA and MD comparisons between different APOE genotypes showed differences in scattered brain clusters (P < 0.01, cluster size = 10). Scattered brain regions showed both higher FA and higher diffusivity in APOE ε2/ε3 compared to APOE ε3/ε3, as well as comparing APOE ε3/ε4 to APOE ε3/ε3. Only RD was decreased in small clusters in APOE ε3/ε4 compared to APOE ε3/ε3 (P < 0.01, cluster size = 10). And AX comparison between APOE ε2/ε3 vs. APOE ε3/ε3 showed more brain regions with higher AX in APOE ε2/ε3 carriers. MD showed similar pattern as of AX.

Furthermore, track-based mean FA stratified by different APOE genotype in majority of fibers demonstrated an incremental consistent pattern (44-24-33-23-34-22 chain, lowest in APOE44 and highest in APOE22 carriers); especially in right cortico-spinal tract and bilateral uncinate fasciculus (**Figure 4**). RD waveforms of 20 ROIs stratified by APOE genotype showed different waveforms than FA, with highest RD in APOE ε2/ε3 isoforms, and lower in APOE ε4+ carriers in all 20 ROIs. Both MD and AX measures showed very similar waveforms as of RD in 20 ROIs.

In addition, 11 out of 26 seed-based fcMRI strength (mean Z-value, with P < 0.001) stratified by different APOE genotype follow an incremental pattern with the 44-24-33-23-34-22 isoform including mean fcMRI seeding from subcortical thalamus (b–e), hypothalamus (f), and task-positive intra-parietal sulcus (a) as well as ventral medial prefrontal cortex; especially the hypothalamus (f) and from the thalamus segment 3 (d) that projected to visual cortex. On the other hand,

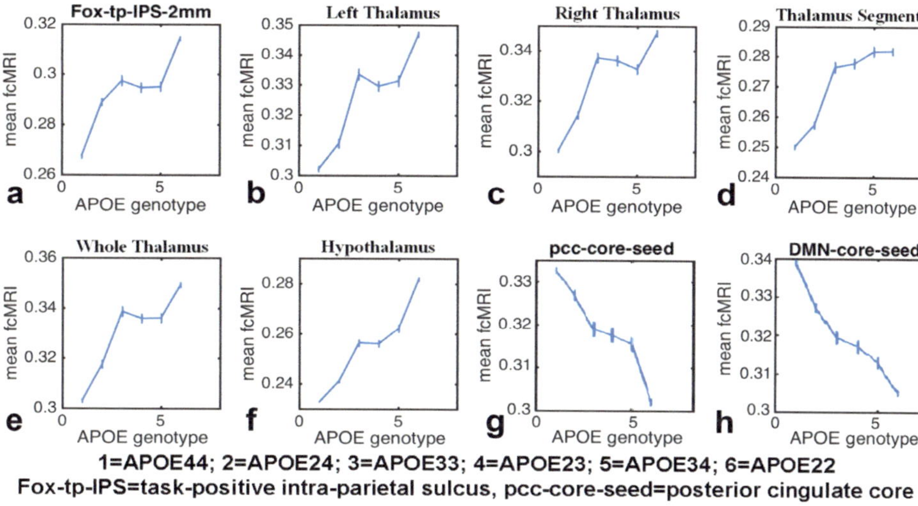

Figure 4.
Effects of APOE genotype on global fcMRI strength of task-positive networks seeding from intra-parietal sulcus (a), thalamus (b,c,d,e) and hypothalamus (f) demonstrated increasing patterns of fcMRI along with the 44-24-33-23-34-22 genotype. On the other hand, decreasing genotypic patterns of resting-state default mode networks (DMN) seeding from the posterior cingulum (g) and core seeds of DMN (h) were observed.

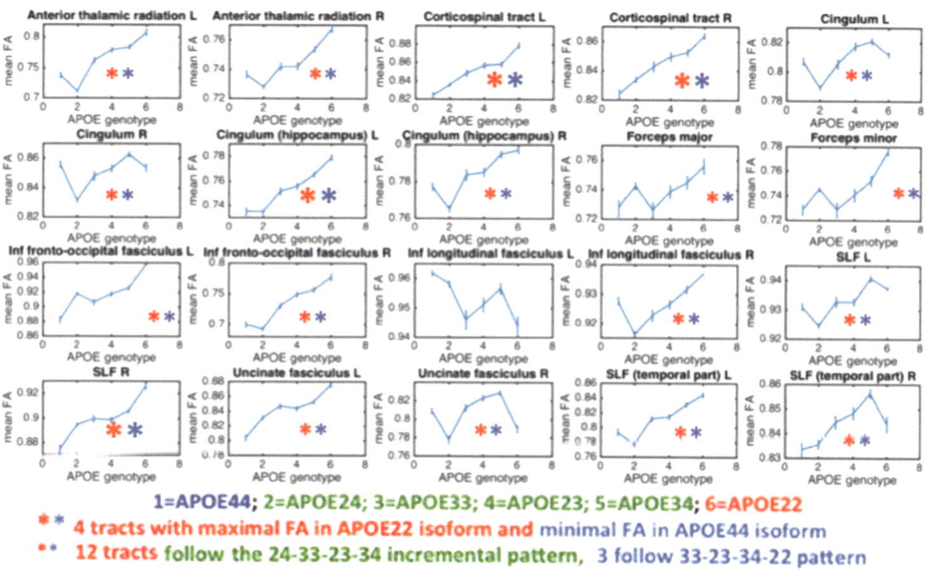

Figure 5.
*APOE genotypic effects on tract-specific DTI mean FA in 20 brain tracts. The mean FA of bilateral corticospinal, left cingulum and right superior longitudinal fasciculus tracts (marked with large **) follow the APOE 44-24-33-23-34 incremental pattern consistently. Inf = inferior; SLF = superior longitudinal fasciculus; L = left; R = right.*

gradual decrement of fcMRI strength with the APOE 44-24-33-23-34-22 genotypic chain of the DMN connecting from the posterior cingulate cortex (PCC) seed (g) and DMN core seed (h) had been observed as well (**Figure 5**).

3.5 fALFF and fcMRI results

As of fALFF, group mean image demonstrated higher fALFF in cortical gray matter with only temporal cortex largely spared (**Figure 6a**). Baseline aging effects

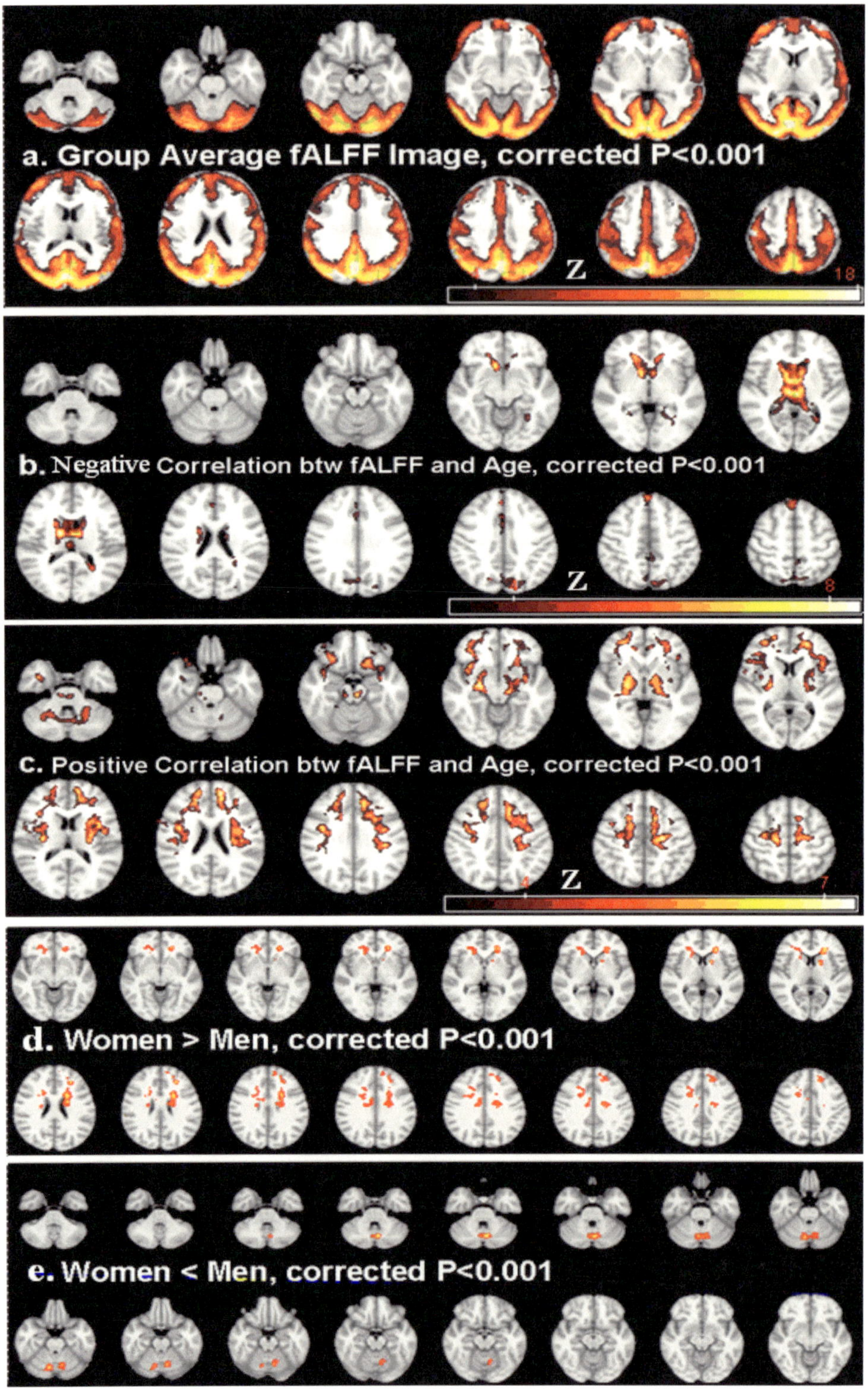

Figure 6.
Functional activity measured with fALFF with group mean (a) (corrected P < 0.001) showing higher fALFF in cortical gray matter with only temporal cortex largely spared. Decreased activity with age in the superior middle frontal and precuneus as well as in the cortical caudate region (b), but increased activity in the cerebellum and bilateral frontal white matter (c) (both cluster corrected P < 0.001) were observed. Women group had higher fALFF Z values in frontal white matter area and small regions in caudate (d), while men group had higher fALFF in cerebellum (e) (both corrected P < 0.001).

demonstrated decreased activity with age in the caudate, superior middle frontal and precuneus regions, but increased activity in the cerebellum and bilateral frontal white matter ($P < 0.001$) (**Figure 6b** and **c**). Average fALFF activity strength over the whole brain demonstrated magnificent aging effects ($r = -0.28$, $P = 0.00001$). Gender comparison showed slight difference with men had lower fALFF than women in small regions of caudate and frontal white matter clusters, but higher activity of men than women in the cerebellum ($P < 0.001$) (**Figure 6d** and **e**). Longitudinal comparison of baseline fALFF and 3 years later showed decreased functional activity in the right inferior parietal lobe and right occipital cortex; accompanied by increased activity in the front eye field region, left superior frontal and left temporal cortices ($P < 0.01$).

3.6 Correlations

LME model performed to available 52 neurocognitive tests at baseline also found significant aging effects ($P < 0.00001$) in almost all tests with worsening cognitive function at age. And similar longitudinal interval effects were found with a smaller significance level for each cognitive test (most $P < 0.001$).

Significant correlations between average Z-value of fcMRI strength in the DMN and neurocognitive tests were found as following: (1) between DMN Z and digital span test (DST) total score ($r = 0.19$, $P < 0.00001$); (2) between average DMN Z and Pegboard dominant (Dom) motor function score ($r = 0.22$, $P < 0.00001$); (3) between average DMN Z and Pegboard non-dominant (NonDom) mean score ($r = 0.17$, $P = 0.00002$); and (4) between average DMN Z and category fluency (FluenCat) test mean score ($r = 0.12$, $P = 0.003$). Interestingly, significant correlations between average DMN Z and graph-theory based resting-state functional network small-worldness properties were found as well, including: (1) between DMN Z and relative local efficiency ($r = 0.15$, $P = 0.0002$); (2) between DMN Z and absolute local efficiency ($r = 0.17$, $P = 0.00002$); (3) between DMN Z and relative global efficiency ($r = 0.09$, $P = 0.02$); (4) between DMN Z and absolute global efficiency ($r = 0.1$, $P = 0.01$); and (5) between DMN Z and small-worldness configuration ($r = 0.15$, $P = 0.0001$). Significant correlations between age and average DMN Z ($r = -0.20$, $P < 0.00001$; $N = 608$) are noted additionally.

Significant correlations between four DTI metrics (FA/MD/AX/MD) and neurocognitive functions were found including California verbal learning test (CVLT), Fluencat, Benton visual retention total errors (BVTOT), Dom and NDom tests that measure visual perception and memory dysfunction, language fluency, communication and social function, speed and accuracy, cognitive flexibility, visual attention, spatial orientation, working memory and executive function, as well as movement speed and motor function domains (most $P < 0.0001$). And correlations were found in all 20 tracts that connect to the whole brain indicating regional and global-wise associations between brain structure connectivity and neurocognitive alterations.

Significant correlations among imaging metrics were found as well including: (1) average whole-brain fALFF (a biomarker for functional activity) Z-value based on resting-state fMRI data and age ($r = -0.28$, $P = 0.00002$); (2) average fALFF Z and mean FA of whole brain ($r = 0.26$, $P = 0.00007$); (3) average DMN Z and mean FA of whole brain ($r = 0.18$, $P = 0.007$); and (4) average DMN Z and mean FA of DMN regions ($r = 0.19$, $P = 0.004$).

4. Discussion and conclusion

One of the main findings of DTI was the decreased FA but increased RD along the age based on both voxel-wise and track-specific analyses at both baseline and longitudinal follow-up visits. Longitudinal data revealed similar rate of change of DTI metrics associated with age and gender as to cross-sectional results, indicating these changes were observable over a very short period (e.g., longitudinal interval of 1–3 years). Especially the significant decreases of FA along the age in most of brain regions suggest that white matter integrity reduces with age. Radial diffusivity (RD) increased with age in the regions that play important roles in memory, visual and motor function such as bilateral thalamic radiations, bilateral somatosensory cortex, visual cortex, anterior and posterior cingulate gyri, middle temporal cortex and hippocampus ($P < 0.01$, cluster size = 10). This suggested that demyelination process that resulted in radial space increases occurred in these brain tracts with age, and was also confirmed with significant reduced fiber-bundles from fornix and parahippocampus, as well as the latest maturation age of the cingulum bundle that was more vulnerable to demyelination and retrograde degeneration [1]. While changes in AX and MD are in two-way: increased AX and MD in some tracts and cortical regions including bilateral thalamic radiation and cingulum bundles, together with decreased AX and MD in some long-distance fasciculus including bilateral corticospinal tract, inferior longitudinal fasciculus and optic radiation. Lower FA and higher RD indicating axonal degeneration have been found in a small sample with similar age range [24, 33]. A few long commissure and association fibers including corpus callosum, cortico-spinal tract, cingulum bundle and superior longitudinal fibers might also undergo Wallerian degeneration [34] with increased RD but decreased AX along the age [1].

Consistent with the current view of neuroplasticity, neuroprotective and compensation roles of fMRI connectivity and activation [35–37], mean fcMRI values from DMN core and PCC core were lowest in the least risky APOE22 isoform, but highest in the most risky APOE44 isoform. And the waveforms of global DMN fcMRI strength decreases from the most to least risky genetic isoforms. However, for the subcortical regions including thalamus and hypothalamus seeds, the fcMRI increases from the expected most risky to least risky genetic isoforms. These changes of divergent waveforms of fcMRI from DMN and subcortical regions had also confirmed the opposite directions of resting-state DMN network and task-positive or attentional-recruitment networks, and might indicate less efficient or over-recruitment of neuronal source usage at most risky APOE44 carriers [38–41]. On the other hand, the DTI metric of FA from majority of fibers demonstrated an incremental consistent pattern from APOE44 to APOE22 carriers, indicating micro-structural integrity was associated positively and tightly with the genotypic functional role of each APOE allele.

Our results of significant imaging quantifications and neurocognitive tests indicate neuronal degeneration, functional disconnectivity as well as white matter deterioration (demyelination, Wallerian degeneration and structural connectivity) at age go parallel with each other, and present together with neurocognitive dysfunction (especially in the domains of memory, cognitive flexibility, visual perception and attention, and executive function). Similar correlation results were found between each tract-specific DTI metric and one-domain neurocognitive test suggest that regional correlations agree with each other, and significant structural connectivity-neurocognitive function correlations remain consistent across the whole brain. Associations between DMN functional connectivity and neurocognitive scores of memory, motor coordination and language social function are expected given the importance of DMN in these domains [42–44]. DMN also represents more global integration function based on the significant correlations between DMN fcMRI and local/global efficiencies of network analysis [45, 46]. Significant correlations were also found between global FA and global functional activity from fALFF; as well as between DMN fcMRI and DMN FA. Scattered longitudinal changes and gender differences of fALFF were found with different patterns from fcMRI (largely decreased DMN but increased DAN regions of fcMRI). However, the spatial distribution pattern of fALFF was mainly in cortical gray matter (significantly higher in occipital, parietal and frontal cortices but with relatively lower activation pattern in temporal cortex). Although fALFF is not a good biomarker due to lack of functional and spatial specialization, it might be used in epoch-related task fMRI study to reflect neuronal activation under task conditions [28].

While our results are consistent with several published articles and are also in agreement with functional and structural connectivity findings [36, 47–50], current study is still limited to the scope of conventional fMRI and DTI sequence with normal aging samples. Further improvement of the technique with acceleration-based fMRI acquisition and multi-shell and multi-b-value DTI [32] as well as validation of our observations using other molecular imaging findings such as amyloid and tau imaging that provide pathological evidence besides the current neuroimaging findings are expected [23, 32, 51, 52]. It had been reported that task-based fMRI data could reflect specific cognitive function such as executive function, high-level cognitive function and communication skill, we expect more correlations could be found between fMRI data and neurocognitive scores in other cognitive domains [53, 54].

In conclusion, different sensitivities of DTI metrics in various brain regions have been observed of the age, gender and genotypic effects. For instance, FA measures showed age effects on white matter integrity across adulthood, with increases in FA through the 30's and 40's and subsequent decreases in middle-age and older adults. Accompanying the decreases of FA along the age in most of brain regions are the radial diffusivity increases that indicates demyelination process with age. AX and MD showed both lower and higher with age in different brain regions, suggesting possible axonal and Wallerian degenerations in these brain regions. We found longitudinal changes in both DTI and fcMRI in regions were similar to those demonstrating cross-sectional effects of age; for instance decreased fcMRI in DMN but increased fcMRI in anti-correlated DAN networks. The APOE genotypic signatures of FA and functional connectivity suggested possible tight associations between myelin/neuronal activation and APOE gene, indicating different roles of APOE alleles on brain structural conductivity, demyelination and neuroplasticity. Taken together, our neuroimaging and correlational neurocognitive results indicate significant and consistent age, gender and APOE genotypic effects on structural and functional connectivity at both baseline and longitudinal short-interval ranges.

Author details

Yongxia Zhou[1,2]

1 Department of Radiology, Columbia University, New York, NY, USA

2 Department of Biomedical Engineering, University of Southern California, Los Angeles, CA, USA

*Address all correspondence to: yongxia.zhou@yahoo.com

References

[1] Zhou Y. Functional Neuroimaging with Multiple Modalities. New York, USA: Nova Publishers; 2016

[2] Huster D, Yao X, Hong M. Membrane protein topology probed by (1) H spin diffusion from lipids using solid-state NMR spectroscopy. Journal of the American Chemical Society. 2002;**124**:874-883

[3] Basser PJ. Inferring microstructural features and the physiological state of tissues from diffusion-weighted images. NMR in Biomedicine. 1995;**8**:333-344

[4] Zhou XJ. Diffusion tensor imaging: Techniques and clinical applications. In: Conference Proceedings: Annual International Conference of the IEEE Engineering in Medicine and Biology Society IEEE Engineering in Medicine and Biology Society Annual Conference. Vol. 7. 2004. pp. 5223-5225

[5] Thiessen JD, Zhang Y, Zhang H, et al. Quantitative MRI and ultrastructural examination of the cuprizone mouse model of demyelination. NMR in Biomedicine. 2013;**26**:1562-1581

[6] Billiet T, Vandenbulcke M, Madler B, et al. Age-related microstructural differences quantified using myelin water imaging and advanced diffusion MRI. Neurobiology of Aging. 2015;**36**:2107-2121

[7] Gazes Y, Bowman FD, Razlighi QR, O'Shea D, Stern Y, Habeck C. White matter tract covariance patterns predict age-declining cognitive abilities. NeuroImage. 2016;**125**:53-60

[8] Sasson E, Doniger GM, Pasternak O, Tarrasch R, Assaf Y. Structural correlates of cognitive domains in normal aging with diffusion tensor imaging. Brain Structure and Function. 2012;**217**:503-515

[9] Agosta F, Dalla Libera D, Spinelli EG, et al. Myeloid microvesicles in cerebrospinal fluid are associated with myelin damage and neuronal loss in mild cognitive impairment and Alzheimer disease. Annals of Neurology. 2014;**76**:813-825

[10] Kochunov P, Glahn DC, Lancaster J, et al. Fractional anisotropy of cerebral white matter and thickness of cortical gray matter across the lifespan. NeuroImage. 2011;**58**:41-49

[11] Horch RA, Gore JC, Does MD. Origins of the ultrashort-T2 1H NMR signals in myelinated nerve: A direct measure of myelin content? Magnetic Resonance in Medicine. 2011;**66**:24-31

[12] Zhou Y. Neuroimaging in Multiple Sclerosis. New York, USA: Nova Publishers; 2017

[13] Bendfeldt K, Kuster P, Traud S, Egger H, Winklhofer S, Mueller-Lenke N, et al. Association of regional gray matter volume loss and progression of white matter lesions in multiple sclerosis—A longitudinal voxel-based morphometry study. NeuroImage. 2009;**45**:60-67

[14] Bjartmar C, Wujek JR, Trapp BD. Axonal loss in the pathology of MS: Consequences for understanding the progressive phase of the disease. Journal of the Neurological Sciences. 2003;**206**:165-171

[15] Bodini B, Khaleeli Z, Cercignani M, Miller DH, Thompson AJ, Ciccarelli O. Exploring the relationship between white matter and gray matter damage in early primary progressive multiple sclerosis: An in vivo study with TBSS and VBM. Human Brain Mapping. 2009;**30**:2852-2861

[16] Kolasa M, Hakulinen U, Helminen M, Hagman S, Raunio M, Rossi M, et al. Longitudinal assessment of clinically

isolated syndrome with diffusion tensor imaging and volumetric MRI. Clinical Imaging. 2015;**39**:207-212

[17] Rocca MA, Preziosa P, Mesaros S, Pagani E, Dackovic J, Stosic-Opincal T, et al. Clinically isolated syndrome suggestive of multiple sclerosis: Dynamic patterns of gray and white matter changes—A 2-year MR imaging study. Radiology. 2016;**278**:841-853

[18] Forn C, Barros-Loscertales A, Escudero J, Benlloch V, Campos S, Antonia Parcet M, et al. Compensatory activations in patients with multiple sclerosis during preserved performance on the auditory N-back task. Human Brain Mapping. 2007;**28**:424-430

[19] Lowe MJ, Beall EB, Sakaie KE, Koenig KA, Stone L, Marrie RA, et al. Resting state sensorimotor functional connectivity in multiple sclerosis inversely correlates with transcallosal motor pathway transverse diffusivity. Human Brain Mapping. 2008;**29**:818-827

[20] Lisak RP. Neurodegeneration in multiple sclerosis: Defining the problem. Neurology. 2007;**68**:S5-S12, discussion S43-54

[21] Yount R, Raschke KA, Biru M, et al. Traumatic brain injury and atrophy of the cingulate gyrus. The Journal of Neuropsychiatry and Clinical Neurosciences. 2002;**14**(4):416-423

[22] Hudak A, Warner M, Marquez de la Plata C, Moore C, Harper C, Diaz-Arrastia R. Brain morphometry changes and depressive symptoms after traumatic brain injury. Psychiatry Research. 2011;**191**(3):160-165

[23] Zhou Y. Neuroimaging in Mild Traumatic Brain Injury. New York, USA: Nova Publishers; 2017

[24] Bender AR, Raz N. Normal-appearing cerebral white matter in healthy adults: Mean change over 2 years and individual differences in change. Neurobiology of Aging. 2015;**36**:1834-1848

[25] McCarrey AC, An Y, Kitner-Triolo MH,Ferrucci L, Resnick SM. Gender differences in cognitive trajectories in clinically normal older adults. Psychology and Aging. 2016;**31**:166-175

[26] Zhou Y, Milham MP, Lui YW, Miles L, Reaume J, Sodickson DK, et al. Default-mode network disruption in mild traumatic brain injury. Radiology. 2002;**265**:882-892

[27] Andrews-Hanna JR, Reidler JS, Sepulcre J, Poulin R, Buckner RL. Functional-anatomic fractionation of the brain's default network. Neuron. 2010;**65**:550-562

[28] Zhou Y, Lui YW, Zuo XN, Milham MP, Reaume J, Grossman RI, et al. Characterization of thalamo-cortical association using amplitude and connectivity of functional MRI in mild traumatic brain injury. Journal of Magnetic Resonance Imaging. 2014;**39**:1558-1568

[29] Zhou Y. Abnormal structural and functional hypothalamic connectivity in mild traumatic brain injury. Journal of Magnetic Resonance Imaging. 2017;**45**:1105-1112

[30] Fox MD, Raichle ME. Spontaneous fluctuations in brain activity observed with functional magnetic resonance imaging. Nature Reviews. Neuroscience. 2007;**8**:700-711

[31] Goh JO, An Y, Resnick SM. Differential trajectories of age-related changes in components of executive and memory processes. Psychology and Aging. 2012;**27**:707-719

[32] Zhou Y. Functional Neuroimaging Methods and Frontiers. New York, USA: Nova Publishers; 2018

[33] Bartzokis G. Age-related myelin breakdown: A developmental model of cognitive decline and Alzheimer's disease. Neurobiology of Aging. 2004;**25**:5-18. author reply 49-62

[34] Kodiweera C, Alexander AL, Harezlak J, McAllister TW, Wu YC. Age effects and gender differences in human brain white matter of young to middle-aged adults: A DTI, NODDI, and q-space study. NeuroImage. 2016;**128**:180-192

[35] Scheinost D, Finn ES, Tokoglu F, et al. Gender differences in normal age trajectories of functional brain networks. Human Brain Mapping. 2015;**36**:1524-1535

[36] Trachtenberg AJ, Filippini N, Ebmeier KP, Smith SM, Karpe F, Mackay CE. The effects of APOE on the functional architecture of the resting brain. NeuroImage. 2012;**59**:565-572

[37] Shu H et al. Opposite neural trajectories of apolipoprotein E 4 and 2 alleles with aging associated with different risks of Alzheimer's disease. Cerebral Cortex. 2016;**26**:1421-1429

[38] Kennedy KM et al. Effects of beta-amyloid accumulation on neural function during encoding across the adult lifespan. NeuroImage. 2012;**62**:1-8. DOI: 10.1016/j.neuroimage

[39] Buckner RL. Memory and executive function in aging and AD: Multiple factors that cause decline and reserve factors that compensate. Neuron. 2004;**44**:195-208

[40] Sala-Llonch R, Bartres-Faz D, Junque C. Reorganization of brain networks in aging: A review of functional connectivity studies. Frontiers in Psychology. 2015;**6**:663

[41] Legon W, Punzell S, Dowlati E, Adams SE, Stiles AB, Moran RJ. Altered prefrontal excitation/inhibition balance and prefrontal output: Markers of aging in human memory networks. Cerebral Cortex. 2016;**26**(11):4315-4326

[42] Raichle ME, Mac Leod AM, Snyder AZ, Powers WJ, Gusnard DA, Shulman GL. A default mode of brain function. Proceedings of the National Academy of Sciences of the United States of America. 2001;**98**:676-682

[43] Buckner RL, Snyder AZ, Shannon BJ, LaRossa G, Sachs R, Fotenos AF, et al. Molecular, structural, and functional characterization of Alzheimer's disease: Evidence for a relationship between default activity, amyloid, and memory. The Journal of Neuroscience. 2005;**25**:7709-7717

[44] Jones DT et al. Age-related changes in the default mode network are more advanced in Alzheimer disease. Neurology. 2011;**77**:1524-1531. DOI: 10.1212/WNL.0b013e318233b33d

[45] Fjell AM, Sneve MH, Storsve AB, Grydeland H, Yendiki A, Walhovd KB. Brain events underlying episodic memory changes in aging: A longitudinal investigation of structural and functional connectivity. Cerebral Cortex. 2016;**26**:1272-1286

[46] Kennedy KM, Rodrigue KM, Bischof GN, Hebrank AC, Reuter-Lorenz PA, Park DC. Age trajectories of functional activation under conditions of low and high processing demands: An adult lifespan fMRI study of the aging brain. NeuroImage. 2015;**104**:21-34

[47] Westlye LT, Reinvang I, Rootwelt H, Espeseth T. Effects of APOE on brain white matter microstructure in healthy adults. Neurology. 2012;**79**:1961-1969

[48] Ward AM, Mormino EC, Huijbers W, Schultz AP, Hedden T, Sperling RA. Relationships between default-mode network connectivity, medial temporal lobe structure, and age-related memory

deficits. Neurobiology of Aging. 2015;**36**:265-272

[49] Zhou J, Greicius MD, Gennatas ED, et al. Divergent network connectivity changes in behavioural variant frontotemporal dementia and Alzheimer's disease. Brain: A Journal of Neurology. 2010;**133**:1352-1367

[50] Bilgel M, An Y, Zhou Y, et al. Individual estimates of age at detectable amyloid onset for risk factor assessment. Alzheimer's & Dementia: The Journal of the Alzheimer's Association. 2015;**36**(8):2333

[51] Scholl M, Lockhart SN, Schonhaut DR, et al. PET imaging of tau deposition in the aging human brain. Neuron. 2016;**89**(5):971-982

[52] Sheline YI, Raichle ME, Snyder AZ, et al. Amyloid plaques disrupt resting state default mode network connectivity in cognitively normal elderly. Biological Psychiatry. 2010;**67**:584-587

[53] Tsvetanov KA, Henson RN, Tyler LK, Razi A, Geerligs L, Ham TE, et al. Extrinsic and intrinsic brain network connectivity maintains cognition across the lifespan despite accelerated decay of regional brain activation. The Journal of Neuroscience. 2016;**36**:3115-3126

[54] Worthy DA, Davis T, Gorlick MA, Cooper JA, Bakkour A, Mumford JA, et al. Neural correlates of state-based decision-making in younger and older adults. NeuroImage. 2015;**130**:13-23

Chapter 2

The Application of Functional Magnetic Resonance Imaging in Neuropathic Pain

Zhi Dou and Liqiang Yang

Abstract

In the past, neuropathic pain has been lacking in ideal imaging research methods, which not only limits our research on the pathogenesis of neuropathic pain but also seriously affects the prognosis of treatments. With the rapid development of fMRI technology, more and more scholars have begun to use fMRI technology in the study of neuropathic pain in recent years. This provides a new idea for revealing the underlining mechanisms of neuropathic pain and improving the clinical treatment concepts. In this chapter, we summarized the recent studies of fMRI in neuropathic pain so that readers can better understand the research status and future research directions.

Keywords: functional magnetic resonance imaging, brain region, brain network, neuropathic pain

1. Introduction

Neuropathic pain (NP) is a common type of pain disease with a prevalence of 1–2% in the total population [1, 2]. Although it is less common than nociceptive pain caused by degeneration of the spine and bones, neuropathic pain is often more severe, accompanied by severe emotional reactions, and the clinical efficacy is not ideal. The problems caused by neuropathic pain in the declined quality of life and the loss of working capacity have caused enormous burdens on patients, families, and our society. The International Association for the Study of Pain (IASP) defines neuropathic pain as "the pain that arises as a direct consequence of a lesion or diseases affecting the somatosensory system." According to the location of the damage to the nervous system, neuropathic pain can be divided into peripheral and central types. Typical symptoms include hyperalgesia, allodynia, spontaneous pain, paresthesia, and other positive signs, as well as negative signs such as sensory loss and shallow reflex disappear [3].

It is now widely accepted that neuropathic pain is caused by a common change in the sensitivity of peripheral and central nervous system signaling. Peripheral mechanisms may include ectopic and spontaneous discharges, pseudo synaptic conduction, changes in ion channel expression, sympathetic neuron sprouting into dorsal root ganglia, and sensitization of nociceptors. The central mechanism also plays an important role in the pathogenesis of neuropathic pain, especially the processing and integration of information in the high-level centers such as the cerebral cortex, brainstem, and cerebellum, which are closely related to the chronic pain and the emergence of many typical symptoms and signs [3]. In the past, studies on the central mechanism of neuropathic pain were mostly limited to clinical observations and animal experiments. However, in recent years, with the development of neuroimaging techniques, especially the maturity of functional magnetic resonance, researchers have been able to explore the structure and function of the brain in multiple levels, providing new ideas for the study of the underlying changes of central nerves system in neuropathic pain.

2. Functional magnetic resonance imaging (fMRI)

Magnetic resonance imaging is an imaging technique based on the principle of nuclear magnetic resonance. According to the difference of research purposes, it can be roughly divided into two categories: structural imaging and functional imaging. The purpose of structure imaging is mainly to study the anatomical structure of brain tissue and the structural fiber connection between different brain regions. The main techniques are conventional brain structure imaging and voxel-based morphological measurement (VBM), diffusion tensor imaging (DTI), etc. VBM can provide regions of interest for brain function changes. DTI can be used to analyze the anatomical basis of functional connectivity in brain regions and therefore belongs to the generalized fMRI. The narrow sense of fMRI mainly refers to a technique for studying brain function activities by monitoring changes in cerebral blood flow. The purpose is to explore the neural activity of each brain region under different physiological or pathological conditions. According to the differences in research methods, it can be divided into task-state fMRI and resting-state fMRI.

2.1 VBM

VBM is a technique for analyzing brain magnetic resonance images at the voxel level. It can quantitatively calculate the changes in local gray and white matter density and volume, so as to accurately display the morphological changes of brain structure. Neuropathic pain can cause changes in the plasticity of the brain structure, such as variation in the gray matter density of the cortex in the brain region. The degree of gray matter density in some brain regions is also related to various clinical indicators such as the length of disease and pain intensity. These changes can be studied with VBM [4].

By tracking follow-up of patients with herpes zoster (HZ), Cao et al. compared the differences in gray matter volume between patients with acute herpes zoster and postherpetic neuralgia (PHN). They found that the PHN brain showed decreased gray matter volume in the frontal lobe, the parietal lobe, and the occipital lobe but increased in the cerebellum and the temporal lobe. These changes may be correlated with HZ-PHN chronification [5]. In several trigeminal neuralgia studies, the reduction of the volume of the anterior cingulate cortex (ACC) and the increase of the volume of the temporal cortex were found. Li et al. also considered that the increase in the volume of the upper and middle gyrus was proportional to the duration of trigeminal neuralgia [6, 7].

2.2 DTI

Modern brain science believes that the human brain is a complex and efficient network called the brain network. Each region of the brain is responsible for relatively independent functions and has a large number of structural and functional connections with each other. The brain network is formed based on this separation and integration principle. White matter fiber bundle is the material basis for connecting the various nodes of the network for information transmission. Any damage to the structure or function of the white matter fiber bundles may affect the information transmission of the brain and cause disease manifestation. DTI is currently the only noninvasive method for effectively observing and tracking white matter fiber bundles. Because of the directionality of the white matter fiber bundles, the internal water molecules are dispersed in a direction-dependent manner, which is called anisotropic. By tracking of the movement direction of water molecules, DTI can reflect the dispersion characteristics of water in white matter fibers and reveal the influence of neuropathic pain on the connection state of brain network structure.

In many DTI studies, trigeminal neuralgia is the most studied type of neuropathic pain. In the case of primary trigeminal neuralgia caused by neurovascular compression, the degree of damage of the trigeminal white matter fiber can be estimated by DTI, thereby assessing the prognosis of microvascular decompression [8]. The diffusion of water molecules from the trigeminal root and root entry zone can help to classify the TN in order to select a more appropriate treatment [9]. In the study of postherpetic neuralgia, researchers also found that there exists altered microstructure integrity of white matter in multiple brain regions in patients with PHN, and these changes increase in size as the duration of the pain increases [10].

2.3 fMRI

Blood oxygenation level-dependent (BOLD) fMRI technique is currently the most widely used fMRI imaging method [11]. The normal functional activity of neurons requires a stable supply of oxygen provided by hemoglobin in the blood, wherein oxyhemoglobin exhibits diamagnetism in the magnetic field due to the shielding effect of oxygen atoms, while deoxyhemoglobin exhibits paramagnetism. In this way, differences in oxygenated blood and deoxygenated magnetic susceptibility can be captured by magnetically sensitive weighted MR images using BOLD fMRI technique [12]. When neurons are excited, the oxygen consumption of these neurons and their surrounding tissue increases, causing a transient decrease in blood oxygen content. This change in the ratio of oxygenated and deoxygenated hemoglobin causes a downward initial tilt angle of the BOLD signal. Due to the continued demand for oxygen, the blood flow there will increase rapidly, and excessive compensation will make the proportion of oxygenated hemoglobin increase and the BOLD signal go up. When the neurons stop exciting and the demand for oxygen is reduced, BOLD will have a negative signal after the stimulus and then gradually return to the baseline. Therefore, by measuring the changes of BOLD signal, fMRI can detect the activation of various regions of the brain and can analyze the temporal correlation of activation or inhibition of different brain regions by simultaneously recording the time series, thereby establishing functional connections of the brain in a specific state [13, 14].

According to the design type of fMRI research, it can be divided into task state and resting state. Task-state fMRI can detect brain regions closely related to certain functions or stimuli by comparing the fMRI images of subjects with and without tasks. It belongs to the study of functional separation of brain regions. By task-state fMRI, a large amount of data has been obtained about the locations and activations of brain regions in neuropathic pain. Resting-state fMRI refers to the data collection when the subject is lying still, the whole body is relaxed, the external stimuli are excluded, and the awake state is maintained. The obtained information is considered to reflect the spontaneous activities in baseline state of the central nervous system. These spontaneous activities not only consume a lot of energy (60–80% of the total energy consumption of the brain) but also have an inherent spatial pattern called the resting brain functional network, which belongs to the study of functional integration between different brain regions of the brain [15, 16]. Studies have shown that many neurologically related diseases, including neuropathic pain, can have a characteristic impact on this resting brain functional network [17, 18], whereas the study of this brain functional network change is more conducive to the clarification of the disease mechanism and the improvement of the diagnosis and treatment level of neuropathic pain [15].

3. fMRI study of the central mechanism of neuropathic pain

3.1 Pain perception in the brain and the process of information transmission

The brain's perception of pain has been one of the most interesting topics in the field of neuroimaging. Since the initial stage of fMRI technology, there have been a large number of related studies. With the in-depth study of the processing and transmission of pain information, the concept of "pain matrix" has gradually formed, which means that pain is achieved through the division of work between multiple regions of the brain, just like a network structure. The pain matrix mainly includes the thalamus, insula, primary somatosensory cortex (S1), secondary somatosensory cortex (S2), anterior cingulate cortex, periaqueductal gray (PAG), amygdala, etc. (**Figure 1**) [20–22]. Significant functional changes will occur in various brain regions within this pain matrix when suffering from acute nociceptive pain [23].

fMRI can be used not only in humans but also in animals such as rats and monkeys. Among these, spared nerve injury (SNI) rats can produce persistent and stable symptoms such as hyperalgesia, allodynia, and spontaneous pain, which are commonly used in the study of neuropathic pain. Komaki et al. studied the resting-state fMRI changes in the SNI rat model and studied the node efficiency of some regions of interest and the functional connections between regions of interest by graph theory. They found that the centrality and node efficiency of the S1 region

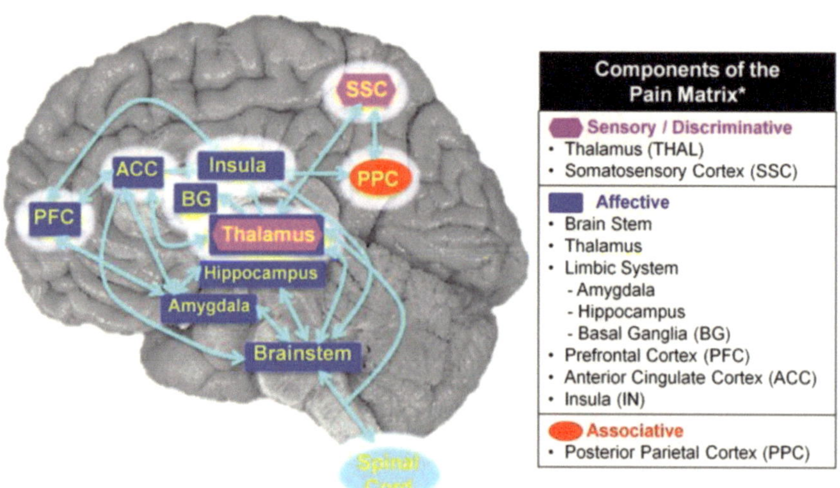

Figure 1.
Schematic diagram of pain matrix [19].

in the opposite side of the injured limb were significantly lower after injury, while the functional connection between the ACC and the posterolateral nucleus of the thalamus was significantly enhanced. This phenomenon may be related to the regulation of secondary nociceptor function by glial cells in the thalamus [24], and mononuclear/macrophage and T lymphocytes may also be involved in [25].

The results of the above studies indicate that although many brain regions involved in pain perception overlap in their respective functions, their functional connections are regularly changing [26]. The lateral thalamus, S2, and insula may be involved in the perception of pain information, and excessive activation of the posterior parietal and prefrontal cortex (PFC) promotes cognitive attention to nociceptive stimuli. Different parts of the ACC are involved in the adaptation or emotional response to pain. Motion control areas (such as basal ganglia, SMA, cerebellum) are involved in the functional regulation of the pain-suppression system and the avoidance behavior of pain. The amygdala plays an important role in the processing of nociceptive information processing and participates in the regulation of medial prefrontal cortex and spinal cord excitability [27, 28]. Abnormal amygdala function is associated with the formation of neuropathic pain, and the destruction of the amygdala can reduce the incidence of neuropathic pain [29]. Through the study of these regular changes, we can deepen the understanding of pain information processing in the brain, and it also helps to define the neurobiological basis of the formation of various typical symptoms of neuropathic pain.

3.2 Chronic process of neuropathic pain

The normal perception of pain and avoidance response is an important physiological protection mechanism. The chronic process of pain is the cause of neuropathic pain and the root of refractory disease. In the past, the understanding of the chronic process of neuropathic pain mostly stayed in the sensitization of nociceptors, the axonal buds of sensory neurons, etc. The understanding of advanced central structures and functional changes in the cerebral cortex was still limited. Nevertheless, fMRI is a powerful tool for studying the process of chronic pain. Both clinical observation and animal experiments have found that chronic process of neuropathic pain is associated with large-scale brain function changes and morphological remodeling [30].

Zhang et al. found that the connection strength of the brain's default network in patients with chronic neuropathic pain was significantly different from that of healthy controls, mainly as the weakening connections in characteristic areas of the default network itself (clamping back in the middle, back, inferior parietal lobule) and motor-related areas (superior parietal lobule, auxiliary sports area) [31]. Hubbard et al.'s task-state fMRI study of SNI rats found that when they stimulated the injured limbs in the injury (4 weeks after surgery), the activity of the contralateral somatosensory cortex (S1, S2), the posterolateral nucleus of the thalamus, and the dorsal striatum was enhanced compared with pre-injury and the control groups, whereas the activity of areas associated with painful emotional responses, such as contralateral insula, medial thalamus, and ipsilateral ACC, was inhibited. Resting-state fMRI study showed an enhanced functional connection between the nucleus accumbens (NAc) and the dorsal striatum. At the same time, molecular biology study found that the expression of dopamine 1A receptor and κ opioid receptor in NAc was downregulated. Moreover, the degree of functional compromise is proportional to the degree of downregulation of dopamine receptor gene expression. Inhibition of NAc's functional activity (injection of lidocaine) significantly reduced pain in SNI model animals [32]. At the late stage of injury (20 weeks after surgery), ACC, prefrontal, insula, basal ganglia, and S1 activity was significantly enhanced, while activity in the medial thalamus and PAG areas was inhibited [33]. It can be seen that the formation of neuropathic pain is related to the inhibition of the function of the descending regulation system of pain [34]. ACC activity is inhibited in the early stages of nerve injury, and with the chronic process of pain, ACC activity is gradually enhanced, which may be related to the unpleasant emotional experience of neuropathic pain [29, 35, 36].

A recent resting-state fMRI study found that several major components of the limbic system, hippocampus, amygdala, striatum, and medial prefrontal cortex, are associated with neuropathic pain formation and maintenance [37]. Although SNI rats showed significant changes of activity degree in some brain regions in the early stage of pain, the functional connection between brain regions was not significantly different from that in rats receiving physiological pain stimulation. It can be considered as a normal response of pain matrix to noxious stimuli. However, with the extension of model establishment time, significant changes in the brain functional network occur, and the remodeled brain network has a specific topology. The vast majority of changes in long-term functional connections (97%) occurred within the edge system, and between the edge system and the nociceptive network, while there were no functional connection changes in the nociceptive network [38]. The limbic system neural network adjusts the reward and punishment, appetite, aversion, etc. to generate emotions and behaviors that can adapt to the pain state, so that the brain network gradually adapts to this pain state and the pain tends to be chronic.

3.3 Hyperalgesia and allodynia

The concept of hyperalgesia and allodynia is often confused, but in fact their formation mechanisms are different. Hyperalgesia refers to a phenomenon in which the pain threshold caused by tissue damage is reduced and the response to noxious stimulation is abnormally enhanced and prolonged. Maihofner et al. found that mechanical pain sensitivity led to abnormal activation of S1, S2, parietal association cortex (PA), insular, superior frontal cortex (SFC), and inferior frontal cortex (IFC) [39], whereas patients with hyperalgesia will have abnormal activation of S1, S2, PA, medial frontal cortex (MFC), ACC, and contralateral SFC and IFC [40]. Zambreanu et al. found that in resting state, patients with no spontaneous pain but hyperalgesia would have abnormal functional activities in multiple regions of the midbrain reticular formation in the brainstem region, namely, nucleus cuneiformis (NCF), rostral superior colliculi (SC), and PAG [41]. The resting-state fMRI of the SNI rat model showed a significant increase in the functional connection between the hippocampus and the striatum, and the intensity was inversely correlated with the mechanical pain threshold of SNI rats.

The clinical manifestation of allodynia is that non-noxious stimuli (such as light touch, mild rubbing, non-noxious cold stimuli) can cause pain, which is a manifestation of "misreading" of somatosensory information. Peripheral sensory nerves are classified into three types: Aβ, Aδ, and C fibers. Normally, the tactile signal is transmitted through the Aβ fiber to the mechanical stimulation zone of the spinal cord. However, in neuropathic pain, Aβ fibers may be abnormally linked to the pain transmission pathway, leading to symptoms such as allodynia [42, 43]. Task-state fMRI is the ideal tool for studying allodynia. Localization and functional connectivity of brain regions associated with allodynia can be achieved by comparing the states of no stimulation, stimulating pain hypersensitivity, and stimulating the same part of the contralateral body. Clinical studies have shown that somatic stimulation signals are amplified by the thalamic and thalamic-parietal circuits, causing excessive activation of the lateral pain sensory system and attention network (posterior parietal lobe). Unlike the response of the thalamic-parietal system, the role of ACC and medial prefrontal lobe in allodynia is more complicated. First, different parts of ACC respond differently to nociceptive stimuli. The central part of ACC was significantly activated during peripheral nerve injury-induced allodynia, whereas there was no significant change in the degree of activation in pain hypersensitivity caused by Wallenberg's lateral infarction. This may be due to the fact that the central part of ACC receives signals from the spinal thalamus bundle and Wallenberg's syndrome causes damage to the spinal thalamic bundle; nevertheless peripheral neuropathic pain does not. However, in most neuropathic pains, whether peripheral or central, the axons of ACC are shown to have a reduced degree of activation when allodynia is induced. The brain regions activated by different stimulating components are also different. Cold and mechanical stimulation can cause significant activation of the prefrontal cortex (PFC) and basal ganglia, and the degree of activation is related to the functional status of ACC [33], and insula signal significantly enhances during stimulation [44].

A similar phenomenon was also found in fMRI study of the SNI animal model by Komaki et al. According to the physiological characteristics of each nerve fiber, the Aβ fiber can be selectively excited by a current of 2000 Hz, 2.2 mA. When the hind paws of normal rats were administered with 2000 Hz, 2.2 mA DC stimulation, it caused only significant activation of the S1 region; however, when the same intensity of current was used to stimulate the pain-sensing hypersensitivity zone of SNI rats, it was found that not only S1, ACC, and thalamus were also significant activated [45].

3.4 Spontaneous pain

Spontaneous pain is generally difficult to study with fMRI. Because it is difficult to obtain a comparison of pain and painlessness in the same patient under clinical conditions, this type of clinical study is still rare. A few studies include spinal cordectomy for cancer pain [46], persistent neuropathic pain before and after local anesthesia [47], and central pain before and after motor cortex stimulation [48]. A common finding of these studies is the reduction in local blood flow in the thalamus, that is, the decrease in thalamic activity, which is restored after pain relief. This depression of lateral thalamic function is found both in peripheral and central neuropathic pain [49].

In the study of trigeminal neuralgia and sphenopalatine neuralgia with typical spontaneous pain characteristics, it was found that the functional connection between the ipsilateral hypothalamus and the contralateral S1 and the ipsilateral wedge was weakened during the pain attack and remission. However, compared with the pain relief period, the functional connection between the hypothalamus and the S1, anterior wedge, and cerebellum is much less during the onset of pain [50].

3.5 Characteristic changes of brain function in different types of neuropathic pain

In addition to the common changes in neuropathic pains, different types of neuropathic pain also have characteristic changes. By studying these changes, it is helpful to clarify its pathogenesis, and it is also possible to screen out specific neuroimaging markers for the diagnosis and evaluation of diseases (**Figure 2**).

Neurovascular compression has long been considered to be the cause of primary trigeminal neuralgia. The 3D TOF MRA and 3D FIESTA sequences can clearly show the positional relationship between the nerves and blood vessels in the root enter zone (REZ) [52–54]. However, nerve compression is not the direct

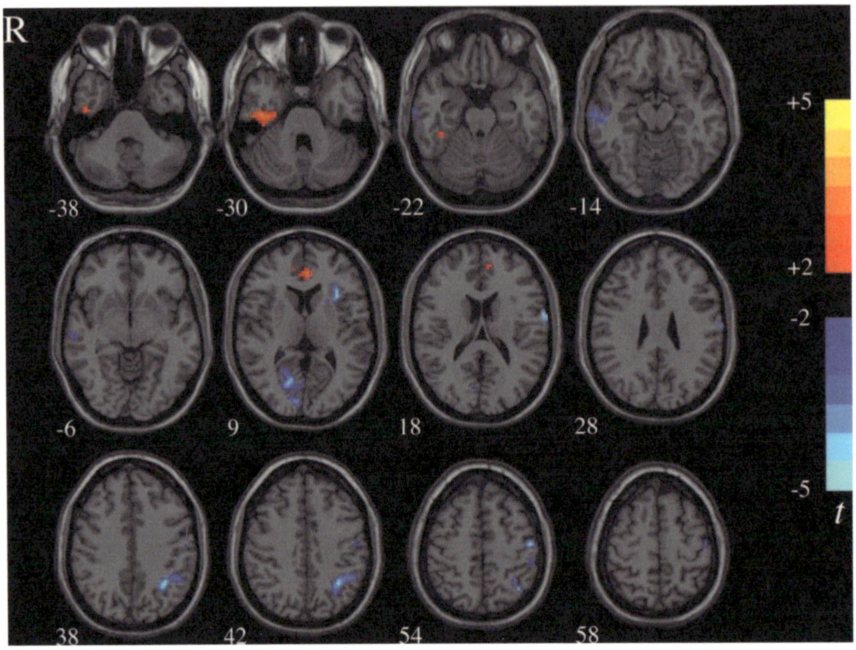

Figure 2.
Characteristic ROIs of trigeminal neuralgia [51].

cause of trigeminal neuralgia. There are also many individuals in the population who have neurological compression but no clinical symptoms of trigeminal neuralgia [55]. Lin et al. found that there were no damage and functional changes in the white matter fibrin myelin or axons in patients with nerve compression but asymptomatic in their DTI study [56]. DeSouza found that the fractional anisotropy (FA) of REZ in patients with trigeminal neuralgia was 22% lower than that of the healthy side and 27% lower than that of healthy controls. Other white matter microstructural measurements of patients such as radial diffusivity (RD), axial diffusivity (AD), and mean diffusivity (MD) were higher than those of healthy controls, indicating demyelinating lesions without axonal injury may be an important factor in the pathogenesis of trigeminal neuralgia [57]. They then compared changes in white matter fiber connections in the REZ region before and after microvascular decompression. It is found that FA, MD, RD, and AD all recovered in the normal direction after treatment and the degree of recovery was proportional to the degree of pain relief [58]. It is suggested that nerve compression by blood vessels is only the inducement of trigeminal neuralgia, and the occurrence and maintenance of pain may be related to abnormal white matter fibers at REZ.

The task-state fMRI conducted by Moisset initially explored the effect of the trigger point of patients with trigeminal neuralgia on brain functional activity. They found that when the pain was onset, spinal trigeminal nucleus (SpV), thalamus, S1, S2, ACC, insular, premotor cortex, motor cortex, frontal nucleus, putamen, etc. were clearly activated in patients with trigger points. In patients without trigger points, the brain regions abovementioned were also activated except SpV, brainstem, and ACC. It can be considered that the structural or functional changes at these three regions may be related to the formation of the trigger point [59]. There are still a small number of studies on resting-state fMRI in patients with trigeminal neuralgia. Athinoula et al. found a weaker functional connection between amygdala and insula and S2 in a comparative study of migraine and trigeminal neuralgia [60].

Wang et al.'s study showed a significant reduction in local consistency activity in the amygdala, hippocampus, and cerebellum in patients with trigeminal neuralgia [61].

The cause of residual limb pain or phantom pain after amputation has been controversial. Some people think that the sudden introduction of nerve afferents from the limbs will cause the expansion or displacement of the sensory cortex, which is called the incompatible remodeling of the cortex [62, 63]. This theory has been proposed for more than 20 years, but it is difficult to be verified before the rise of fMRI technology [64, 65]. Lotze et al. conducted a task-state fMRI study and found that cortical remodeling in patients with phantom limb pain is not limited to S1 but also includes some auxiliary sports areas [66]. For example, when the lips move, the activation degree of the representative region of the broken limb in M1 is also significantly enhanced, indicating that the lip represents region expands and displaces to the cortex of broken limb [67]. Moreover, the degree of displacement of the cortex to the representative area of the isolated limb is positively correlated with the degree of pain [68]. After mirror therapy, cortical displacement can be partially restored, and the pain intensity can be reduced [69].

Cauda et al. found that the functional connections between the ventral posterior nucleus (VP) and the medial dorsal nucleus (MD) and the cerebral cortex were weakened in patients with diabetic peripheral neuropathy [70]. Cifre observed a weakened connection between resting thalamus and insula in patients with fibromyalgia [71]. In patients with postherpetic neuralgia, the reward circuit consisting of the striatum, prefrontal cortex, amygdala, and hippocampus and the circuits composed of striatum, thalamus, and insular leaves have very close functional connection [72]. With the advancement of fMRI data analysis methods and machine learning techniques, these seemingly cluttered functional connectivity features are highly likely to be used as neuroimaging markers for the diagnosis of neuropathic pain. In other studies of nervous system diseases, some scholars have successfully used fMRI technology to construct a resting brain functional network model for patients with Alzheimer's disease. And with the using of multimode variable analysis method, the sensitivity and specificity of early screening of Alzheimer's disease in the general population is up to 90% [73].

4. The value of fMRI in the clinical treatment of neuropathic pain

In the past, the examination and evaluation of neuropathic pain relied mainly on medical history, symptoms, and signs and lacked tools for quantitative assessment. Even with the von Frey fiber test, the same stimulation site and strength often result in a lack of consistency [74]. The reason is that the activity of the nerve is disturbed by many factors. Inclusion of peripheral and central sensitization, genetics, cognition, and emotional response during testing will affect the signal transmission of noxious stimuli to the painful sensation area of the brain [75]. In addition, the subjective tendencies of participants and examiners may also cause serious bias. However, fMRI technology may provide us with qualitative and quantitative observations [76]. For example, PoCG's corresponding somatosensory representative area can help clinicians determine the pain site, and the degree of activation can also reflect the intensity of pain [51]. The local activity consistency of rostralanterior part of ACC in patients with postherpetic neuralgia was significantly correlated with the anxiety and depression scores [77, 78].

fMRI can also be used to observe the effects of treatments on brain function or to assess the therapeutic effects of neuropathic pain. For example, after the application of opioids to achieve pain relief, an increase in ACC activation can be found. Thalamic electrical stimulation can significantly increase the activation of the rostralanterior part of ACC and the basal part of frontal cortex. These two sites are generally in a state of functional inhibition in patients with chronic neuropathic pain. A study of drug therapy for trigeminal neuralgia has shown that lamotrigine can reduce the pain level of patients by reducing the excitability of the prefrontal, parietal, and temporal lobe and inhibit allodynia [79].

As a method for treating neuropathic pain, neuromodulation technology has been applied for decades. However, whether it is invasive spinal cord electrical stimulation, deep brain stimulation, or noninvasive transcranial magnetic stimulation, there is a problem of inefficiency. The reason may be due to individual differences in the effects of disease on the brain functional network. fMRI can accurately capture the brain regions with abnormal functions and combine the analysis of functional connections in the brain to determine the regions of interest for neuromodulation, which is used to guide the target area of transcranial magnetic stimulation or the placement of epidural stimulation electrodes [80, 81]. It is helpful to improve the efficacy of neuromodulation techniques.

5. Limitations and future direction of fMRI research in NP

Most of the previous studies were limited by the fMRI data analysis method. They can only analyze for a single factor, or only focus on brain regions or functional connections with significant differences, while ignoring the complexity and synergy of the brain function network as a whole structure. And the conclusions drawn lack clinical utility and provide limited assistance in the diagnosis and prediction of diseases.

In recent years, with the increasing maturity of machine learning technology, machine learning and pattern recognition technology are being used more and more for fMRI data analysis. By using machine learning technology to process the massive characteristic data generated by fMRI, multiple dimensions such as gray matter volume, diffusion of water molecules, and functional connectivity can be used simultaneously [82]. In the future, this research method of overall analysis of brain function networks can realize pattern recognition of different disease states. It can make fMRI technology better serve the clinic and provide assistance for the diagnosis and prognosis analysis of neuropathic pain.

6. Conclusion

A large number of brain regions associated with neuropathic pain have been discovered by fMRI technology, and there has been some data accumulation for changes in functional connectivity between brain regions. However, how to analyze and process these fMRI data and make a reasonable explanation for better understanding the underlying disease mechanism as well as treatment improvement is the key to further expand the value of fMRI application in the future.

Author details

Zhi Dou* and Liqiang Yang
Department of Pain Management, Xuanwu Hospital, Capital Medical University, Beijing, China

*Address all correspondence to: douzhi@xwhosp.org

References

[1] Jensen TS, Gottrup H, Sindrup SH, et al. The clinical picture of neuropathic pain. European Journal of Pharmacology. 2001;**429**(1-3):1-11

[2] Chong MS, Bajwa ZH. Diagnosis and treatment of neuropathic pain. Journal of Pain and Symptom Management. 2003;**25**(5 Suppl):S4-S11

[3] Vranken JH. Elucidation of pathophysiology and treatment of neuropathic pain. Central Nervous System Agents in Medicinal Chemistry. 2012;**12**(4):304-314

[4] Henry DE, Chiodo AE, Yang W. Central nervous system reorganization in a variety of chronic pain states: A review. PM & R : The Journal of Injury, Function, and Rehabilitation. 2011;**3**(12):1116-1125

[5] Cao S, Qin B, Zhang Y, et al. Herpes zoster chronification to postherpetic neuralgia induces brain activity and grey matter volume change. American Journal of Translational Research. 2018;**10**(1):184-199

[6] Wang Y, Cao DY, Remeniuk B, et al. Altered brain structure and function associated with sensory and affective components of classic trigeminal neuralgia. Pain. 2017;**158**(8):1561-1570

[7] Li M, Yan J, Li S, et al. Reduced volume of gray matter in patients with trigeminal neuralgia. Brain Imaging and Behavior. 2017;**11**(2):486-492

[8] Chai W, You C, Zhang W, et al. Diffusion tensor imaging of microstructural alterations in the trigeminal nerve due to neurovascular contact/compression. Acta Neurochirurgica. 2019;**161**(7):1407-1413

[9] Willsey MS, Collins KL, Conrad EC, et al. Diffusion tensor imaging reveals microstructural differences between subtypes of trigeminal neuralgia. Journal of Neurosurgery. 2019;**6**(19): 1-7

[10] Chen F, Chen F, Shang Z, et al. White matter microstructure degenerates in patients with postherpetic neuralgia. Neuroscience Letters. 2017;**656**:152-157

[11] Ogawa S, Lee TM, Nayak AS, et al. Oxygenation-sensitive contrast in magnetic resonance image of rodent brain at high magnetic fields. Magnetic Resonance in Medicine. 1990;**14**(1):68-78

[12] Logothetis NK. The neural basis of the blood-oxygen-level-dependent functional magnetic resonance imaging signal. Philosophical Transactions of the Royal Society of London. Series B, Biological Sciences. 2002;**357**(1424):1003-1037

[13] Ogawa S, Lee TM, Kay AR, et al. Brain magnetic resonance imaging with contrast dependent on blood oxygenation. Proceedings of the National Academy of Sciences of the United States of America. 1990;**87**(24):9868-9872

[14] Ogawa S, Menon RS, Tank DW, et al. Functional brain mapping by blood oxygenation level-dependent contrast magnetic resonance imaging. A comparison of signal characteristics with a biophysical model. Biophysical Journal. 1993;**64**(3):803-812

[15] Lu H, Yuping N. When neuroscience meets network thinking: A new perspective on brain disorders. Chinese Journal of Neuromedicines. 2014, 2014;**13**(12):1292-1296

[16] Dezhong Y, Luo C, Xu L, et al. Neuroimaging and brain connectome. Chinese Journal of Biomedical Engineering. 2011;**30**(1):6-10

[17] Rubinov M, Sporns O. Weight-conserving characterization of complex functional brain networks. NeuroImage. 2011;**56**(4):2068-2079

[18] Bassett DS, Bullmore ET. Human brain networks in health and disease. Current Opinion in Neurology. 2009;**22**(4):340-347

[19] Melzack R. Evolution of the neuromatrix theory of pain. The Prithvi Raj lecture: Presented at the third World Congress of World Institute of Pain, Barcelona 2004. Pain Practice. 2005;**5**(2):85-94

[20] Wager TD, Atlas LY, Lindquist MA, et al. An fMRI-based neurologic signature of physical pain. The New England Journal of Medicine. 2013;**368**(15):1388-1397

[21] Davis KD, Taylor SJ, Crawley AP, et al. Functional MRI of pain- and attention-related activations in the human cingulate cortex. Journal of Neurophysiology. 1997;**77**(6):3370-3380

[22] Nakao A, Takahashi Y, Nagase M, et al. Role of capsaicin-sensitive C-fiber afferents in neuropathic pain-induced synaptic potentiation in the nociceptive amygdala. Molecular Pain. 2012;**8**:51

[23] Thompson SJ, Bushnell MC. Rodent functional and anatomical imaging of pain. Neuroscience Letters. 2012;**520**(2):131-139

[24] Zhao P, Waxman SG, Hains BC. Modulation of thalamic nociceptive processing after spinal cord injury through remote activation of thalamic microglia by cysteine cysteine chemokine ligand 21. The Journal of Neuroscience. 2007;**27**(33):8893-8902

[25] Wei XH, Zang Y, Wu CY, et al. Peri-sciatic administration of recombinant rat TNF-alpha induces mechanical allodynia via upregulation of TNF-alpha in dorsal root ganglia and in spinal dorsal horn: The role of NF-kappa B pathway. Experimental Neurology. 2007;**205**(2):471-484

[26] Maihofner C, Nickel FT, Seifert F. Neuropathic pain and neuroplasticity in functional imaging studies. Schmerz. 2010;**24**(2):137-145

[27] Baabor MG, Perez-Limonte L. Percutaneous balloon compression of the gasserian ganglion for the treatment of trigeminal neuralgia: Personal experience of 206 patients. Acta Neurochirurgica. Supplement. 2011;**108**:251-254

[28] Bird GC, Lash LL, Han JS, et al. Protein kinase A-dependent enhanced NMDA receptor function in pain-related synaptic plasticity in rat amygdala neurones. The Journal of Physiology. 2005;**564**(3):907-921

[29] Hashmi JA, Baliki MN, Huang L, et al. Shape shifting pain: Chronification of back pain shifts brain representation from nociceptive to emotional circuits. Brain. 2013;**136**(9):2751-2768

[30] Apkarian AV, Baliki MN, Geha PY. Towards a theory of chronic pain. Progress in Neurobiology. 2009;**87**(2):81-97

[31] Hua Z, Hao W, Duoduo L, et al. Default mode network altered in chronic pain caused by cervical spondylosis. Chinese Journal of Rehabilitation Theory and Practice. 2015;**21**(1):69-73

[32] Chang PC, Pollema-Mays SL, Centeno MV, et al. Role of nucleus accumbens in neuropathic pain: Linked multi-scale evidence in the rat transitioning to neuropathic pain. Pain. 2014;**155**(6):1128-1139

[33] Hubbard CS, Khan SA, Xu S, et al. Behavioral, metabolic and functional brain changes in a rat model of chronic neuropathic pain: A longitudinal MRI study. NeuroImage. 2015;**107**:333-344

[34] Maarrawi J, Mertens P, Peyron R, et al. Functional exploration for neuropathic pain. Advances and Technical Standards in Neurosurgery. 2011;**37**:25-63

[35] Davis KD, Taylor KS, Anastakis DJ. Nerve injury triggers changes in the brain. The Neuroscientist. 2011;**17**(4):407-422

[36] Vertes RP. Interactions among the medial prefrontal cortex, hippocampus and midline thalamus in emotional and cognitive processing in the rat. Neuroscience. 2006;**142**(1):1-20

[37] Berger SE, Baria AT, Baliki MN, et al. Risky monetary behavior in chronic back pain is associated with altered modular connectivity of the nucleus accumbens. BMC Research Notes. 2014;7:739

[38] Baliki MN, Chang PC, Baria AT, et al. Resting-sate functional reorganization of the rat limbic system following neuropathic injury. Scientific Reports. 2014;**4**:6186

[39] Maihofner C, Schmelz M, Forster C, et al. Neural activation during experimental allodynia: A functional magnetic resonance imaging study. The European Journal of Neuroscience. 2004;**19**(12):3211-3218

[40] Maihofner C, Handwerker HO. Differential coding of hyperalgesia in the human brain: A functional MRI study. NeuroImage. 2005;**28**(4): 996-1006

[41] Zambreanu L, Wise RG, Brooks JC, et al. A role for the brainstem in central sensitisation in humans. Evidence from functional magnetic resonance imaging. Pain. 2005;**114**(3):397-407

[42] Komori K, Nonaka T, Okada A, et al. Absence of mechanical allodynia and Abeta-fiber sprouting after sciatic nerve injury in mice lacking membrane-type 5 matrix metalloproteinase. FEBS Letters. 2004;**557**(1-3):125-128

[43] Ji RR, Kohno T, Moore KA, et al. Central sensitization and LTP: Do pain and memory share similar mechanisms? Trends in Neurosciences. 2003;**26**(12):696-705

[44] Becerra L, Morris S, Bazes S, et al. Trigeminal neuropathic pain alters responses in CNS circuits to mechanical (brush) and thermal (cold and heat) stimuli. The Journal of Neuroscience. 2006;**26**(42):10646-10657

[45] Komaki Y, Hikishima K, Shibata S, et al. Functional brain mapping using specific sensory-circuit stimulation and a theoretical graph network analysis in mice with neuropathic allodynia. Scientific Reports. 2016;**6**:37802

[46] Di Piero V, Jones AK, Iannotti F, et al. Chronic pain: A PET study of the central effects of percutaneous high cervical cordotomy. Pain. 1991;**46**(1):9-12

[47] Hsieh JC, Belfrage M, Stone-Elander S, et al. Central representation of chronic ongoing neuropathic pain studied by positron emission tomography. Pain. 1995;**63**(2):225-236

[48] Garcia-Larrea L, Peyron R, Mertens P, et al. Electrical stimulation of motor cortex for pain control: A combined PET-scan and electrophysiological study. Pain. 1999;**83**(2):259-273

[49] Peyron R, Garcia-Larrea L, Gregoire MC, et al. Haemodynamic brain responses to acute pain in humans: Sensory and attentional networks. Brain. 1999;**122**(Pt 9):1765-1780

[50] Yang FC, Chou KH, Fuh JL, et al. Altered hypothalamic functional connectivity in cluster headache: A longitudinal resting-state functional

MRI study. Journal of Neurology, Neurosurgery, and Psychiatry. 2015;**86**(4):437-445

[51] Dou Z, Zhang X, Yang L, et al. Alternation of regional homogeneity in trigeminal neuralgia after percutaneous radiofrequency thermocoagulation: A resting state fMRI study. Medicine (Baltimore). 2016;**95**(42):e5193

[52] Montano N, Conforti G, Di Bonaventura R, et al. Advances in diagnosis and treatment of trigeminal neuralgia. Therapeutics and Clinical Risk Management. 2015;**11**:289-299

[53] Maarbjerg S, Wolfram F, Gozalov A, et al. Significance of neurovascular contact in classical trigeminal neuralgia. Brain. 2015;**138**(2):311-319

[54] Docampo J, Gonzalez N, Munoz A, et al. Neurovascular study of the trigeminal nerve at 3 t MRI. The Neuroradiology Journal. 2015;**28**(1):28-35

[55] Zakrzewska JM, Linskey ME. Trigeminal neuralgia. BMJ. 2014;**348**:474-483

[56] Lin W, Chen YL, Zhang QW. Vascular compression of the trigeminal nerve in asymptomatic individuals: A voxel-wise analysis of axial and radial diffusivity. Acta Neurochirurgica. 2014;**156**(3):577-580

[57] DeSouza DD, Hodaie M, Davis KD. Abnormal trigeminal nerve microstructure and brain white matter in idiopathic trigeminal neuralgia. Pain. 2014;**155**(1):37-44

[58] DeSouza DD, Davis KD, Hodaie M. Reversal of insular and microstructural nerve abnormalities following effective surgical treatment for trigeminal neuralgia. Pain. 2015;**156**(6):1112-1123

[59] Moisset X, Villain N, Ducreux D, et al. Functional brain imaging of trigeminal neuralgia. European Journal of Pain. 2011;**15**(2):124-131

[60] Hadjikhani N, Ward N, Boshyan J, et al. The missing link: Enhanced functional connectivity between amygdala and visceroceptive cortex in migraine. Cephalalgia. 2013;**33**(15):1264-1268

[61] Wang Y, Zhang X, Guan Q, et al. Altered regional homogeneity of spontaneous brain activity in idiopathic trigeminal neuralgia. Neuropsychiatric Disease and Treatment. 2015;**11**:2659-2666

[62] Flor H. Cortical reorganisation and chronic pain: Implications for rehabilitation. Journal of Rehabilitation Medicine. 2003;**5**(41):66-72

[63] Foell J, Bekrater-Bodmann R, Diers M, et al. Mirror therapy for phantom limb pain: Brain changes and the role of body representation. European Journal of Pain. 2014;**18**(5):729-739

[64] Flor H, Elbert T, Knecht S, et al. Phantom-limb pain as a perceptual correlate of cortical reorganization following arm amputation. Nature. 1995;**375**(6531):482-484

[65] Jutzeler CR, Curt A, Kramer JL. Relationship between chronic pain and brain reorganization after deafferentation: A systematic review of functional MRI findings. NeuroImage. Clinical. 2015;**9**:599-606

[66] Dettmers C, Adler T, Rzanny R, et al. Increased excitability in the primary motor cortex and supplementary motor area in patients with phantom limb pain after upper limb amputation. Neuroscience Letters. 2001;**307**(2):109-112

[67] Lotze M, Flor H, Grodd W, et al. Phantom movements and pain. An fMRI

study in upper limb amputees. Brain. 2001;**124**(11):2268-2277

[68] Gustin SM, Wrigley PJ, Henderson LA, et al. Brain circuitry underlying pain in response to imagined movement in people with spinal cord injury. Pain. 2010;**148**(3):438-445

[69] Diers M, Christmann C, Koeppe C, et al. Mirrored, imagined and executed movements differentially activate sensorimotor cortex in amputees with and without phantom limb pain. Pain. 2010;**149**(2):296-304

[70] Cauda F, Sacco K, D'Agata F, et al. Low-frequency BOLD fluctuations demonstrate altered thalamocortical connectivity in diabetic neuropathic pain. BMC Neuroscience. 2009;**10**:138

[71] Cifre I, Sitges C, Fraiman D, et al. Disrupted functional connectivity of the pain network in fibromyalgia. Psychosomatic Medicine. 2012;**74**(1):55-62

[72] Liu J, Hao Y, Du M, et al. Quantitative cerebral blood flow mapping and functional connectivity of postherpetic neuralgia pain: A perfusion fMRI study. Pain. 2013;**154**(1):110-118

[73] Craddock RC, Holtzheimer PE, Hu XP, et al. Disease state prediction from resting state functional connectivity. Magnetic Resonance in Medicine. 2009;**62**(6):1619-1628

[74] Tracey I. Getting the pain you expect: Mechanisms of placebo, nocebo and reappraisal effects in humans. Nature Medicine. 2010;**16**(11):1277-1283

[75] Basbaum AI, Bautista DM, Scherrer G, et al. Cellular and molecular mechanisms of pain. Cell. 2009;**139**(2):267-284

[76] Bosshard SC, Baltes C, Wyss MT, et al. Assessment of brain responses to innocuous and noxious electrical forepaw stimulation in mice using BOLD fMRI. Pain. 2010;**151**(3):655-663

[77] Vogt BA, Finch DM, Olson CR. Functional heterogeneity in cingulate cortex: The anterior executive and posterior evaluative regions. Cerebral Cortex. 1992;**2**(6):435-443

[78] Vogt BA, Sikes RW. The medial pain system, cingulate cortex, and parallel processing of nociceptive information. Progress in Brain Research. 2000;**122**:223-235

[79] Scrivani S, Wallin D, Moulton EA, et al. A fMRI evaluation of lamotrigine for the treatment of trigeminal neuropathic pain: Pilot study. Pain Medicine. 2010;**11**(6):920-941

[80] De Ridder D, Vanneste S, Van Laere K, et al. Chasing map plasticity in neuropathic pain. World Neurosurgery. 2013;**80**(6):901-905

[81] De Ridder D, Elgoyhen AB, Romo R, et al. Phantom percepts: Tinnitus and pain as persisting aversive memory networks. Proceedings of the National Academy of Sciences of the United States of America. 2011;**108**(20):8075-8080

[82] Glasser MF, Coalson TS, Robinson EC, et al. A multi-modal parcellation of human cerebral cortex. Nature. 2016;**536**(7615):171-178

Section 2

Nuclear Medicine PET/CT Imaging and Applications

Chapter 3

The Ionizing Radiation Interaction with Matter, the X-ray Computed Tomography Imaging, the Nuclear Medicine SPECT, PET and PET-CT Tomography Imaging

Evangelos Gazis

Abstract

The mechanism of the ionizing radiation interaction with matter is described for heavy charged particles, electrons and photons. Those effects causing energy loss of the radiation with sequential effects of absorption or attenuation are presented. The features of some characteristic detector systems with the relative electronics and the data acquisition system (DAQ) are presented. Those detectors are related with the medical imaging sensor systems. The characteristics of the medical imaging process of the X-ray and nuclear imaging with SPECT, PET and the combination of PET-CT are presented. The computed X-ray tomography, called CT, and the nuclear medicine tomography are presented, implementing the most of the previous parts, as they are defined in PET and SPECT imaging plus the combination of PET with CT the PET-CT.

Keywords: ionizing radiation, X-ray imaging, nuclear medicine, PET, SPECT, PET-CT imaging

1. Introduction

The approach of this chapter is to cover physical principles of the interaction mechanisms of the ionizing radiation, the instrumental detector design and the relative electronics with the data acquisition setup, the image reconstruction techniques, and clinical applications of the imaging techniques most commonly used in clinical medicine as well as in academic research. It starts with the ionizing radiation interaction with matter for various particles and the properties then, the X-ray computed tomography, finishing with the nuclear medicine imaging with SPECT, PET and PET-CT imaging.

2. The ionizing radiation interaction with matter

Unstable nuclei can emit a variety of electrically charged and neutral, particles as well as electromagnetic radiation known as γ-rays (energetic photons).

The best-known particle emission modes are the α-decay, in which a Helium nucleus is produced, and β-decay where an energetic electron e− (or a positron, e+) and an anti-neutrino (or a neutrino) are created. All these emissions are generically referred to as nuclear radiation. Their interaction with matter may occur via the electromagnetic, the strong or the week nuclear forces. An important issue in studying the passage of energetic nuclear radiation through matter is in understanding the transfer of energy produced. Energy transfer mechanisms depend on a number of factors, such as the type of radiation and its energy, as well as the physical properties of the irradiated material. Electrically charged particles, and γ-rays, of nuclear origin interact with highest probability with atomic excitation and ionization. In many of those processes, secondary electrons are produced which spread the energy deposition away from the primary interaction region. Measuring the effects of radiation on matter and finding out the relationship between them and the energy lost by the original radiation is the basis of all nuclear detection methods. When dealing with leaving matter, the biological impacts of such phenomena are the subject of much concern and study [1–4].

2.1 Interaction of alpha particles

The alpha particles (nuclei of Helium) have two protons and two neutrons bound together. Their mass is relatively large and carries a double positive charge. Alpha particles are commonly spontaneously emitted by the heavy radioactive nuclei occurring in the nature (Uranium, Thorium or Radium), as well as the transuranic elements (Neptunium, Plutonium or Americium). The high mass and charge of an alpha particle, relative to other forms of nuclear radiation, causes its greater ionization power and poorer ability to penetrate matter. A piece of paper can stop them. They travel only a few centimeters but deposit all their energies along their short paths.

2.1.1 Stopping power

The alpha charged particles passing through matter lose kinetic energy by excitation of bound electrons and by ionization. The maximum transferable kinetic energy to an electron depends on the mass m_0 and the momentum of the incident alpha particle. Given the momentum of the incident particle, $p = \gamma m_0 \beta c$, where γ is the Lorentz factor ($= E/m_0c^2$), $\beta c = v$ the velocity, and m_0 the rest mass; then the maximum transferable energy to electron with mass m_e is

$$E_{kin}^{max} = \frac{2m_e c^2 \beta^2 \gamma^2}{1 + 2\gamma m_e/m_0 + (m_e/m_0)^2} = \frac{2m_e p^2}{m_0^2 + m_e^2 + 2m_e E/c^2} \qquad (1)$$

For low energies:

$$2\gamma m_e/m_0 \ll 1 \qquad (2)$$

and under the assumption that the incident alpha particles are heavier than electrons ($m_0 > m_e$) Eq. (1) can be approximated by

$$E_{kin}^{max} \approx 2m_e c^2 \beta^2 \gamma^2 \qquad (3)$$

The Energy loss for heavy charged particle per unit length [dE/dx], called stopping power, is given by

$$\frac{dE}{dx} \propto \frac{Z^2}{\beta^2} \ln\left(a\beta^2\gamma^2\right) \tag{4}$$

Z = atomic number of the material, a = material-dependent constant.

The trajectory of the charged alpha particle is unchanged after scattering, as in the **Figure 1**.

2.1.2 Bethe-Bloch relation

Therefore, the mean energy loss for 'heavy' charged particles through the matter is given by the Bethe and Bloch formula [5–8].

$$-\left\langle \frac{dE}{dx} \right\rangle = 2\pi N_A r_e^2 m_e c^2 \rho \frac{Z}{A} \frac{z^2}{\beta^2} \left[\ln\left(\frac{2m_e c^2 \beta^2 \gamma^2}{I^2} \right) - 2\beta^2 - \delta(\beta\gamma) \right] \tag{5}$$

Fundamental constants: r_e = classical radius of electron, N_A = Avogadro's number.

Absorber medium: I = mean ionization potential, approximately $I = 16Z^{0.9}$ if $Z > 1$, Z = atomic number of absorber, A = atomic weight of absorber, ρ = density of absorber, δ = density correction, z = atomic number of the incident particle.

2.1.3 Range of alpha particles

A heavy charged particle, such as an alpha particle, has a fairly definite range in a gas, liquid, or solid. The particle loses energy, primarily by the excitation and ionization of atoms in its path, occurs in a large number of small increments. The alpha particle has such a large momentum that its direction is not changed appreciably during the slowing processes. Eventually it loses all its kinetic energy and comes to rest. The distance traversed is called the range, and depends on the energy of the alpha particle, the atom density in the material traversed, and the atomic number and average ionization potential of the atoms comprising this material. Integrate over energy loss from the total energy T to the zero, it is obtained the alpha particles range:

$$R(T) = \int_0^T \left[-\frac{dE}{dx} \right]^{-1} dE \tag{6}$$

A plot of the specific ionization (number of ions formed per unit distance of beam path) versus distance from the alpha particle source for a beam of alpha particles is called a Bragg curve, should have the shape shown in **Figure 2**.

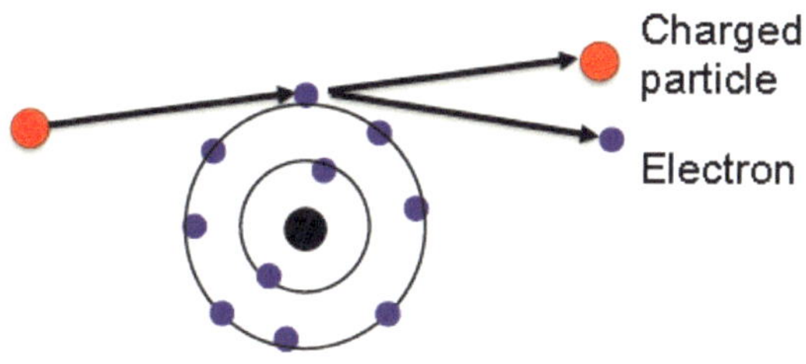

Figure 1.
The alpha particle trajectory remains unchanged after ionizing the atom passing through.

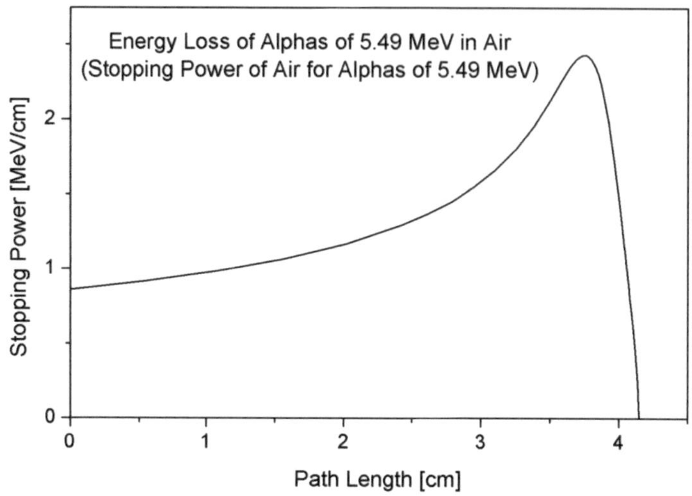

Figure 2.
The alpha particles range in air. The trajectory called Bragg curve has the characteristic peak as the majority of the particles energy is deposited at the last stage of the curve.

2.2 Interaction of electrons and positrons

The interaction of electrons with the matter follows the same mechanism of the charged particles with the absorbed material; taking into account that the incident and target electron have same mass m_e, so the incident and scattering electrons are identical and undistinguishable particles. Electrons as incident particles, however, play a special role in the treatment of the energy loss as the total energy loss of electrons even at low energies (MeV range) is influenced by bremsstrahlung processes. In addition, the ionization loss requires different treatment because the energy-transfer probability must be interpreted in a different way. One electron after the collision receives the energy E_{kin} and the other electron the rest of the energy $E - m_e c^2 - E_{kin}$, where E is the total energy of the incident electron.

The positrons have similar ionization loss as those of the electrons, having these particles are of equal mass, but not identical charge. Under the assumption that the positrons are antiparticles of electrons, there is, however, an additional consideration: if positrons come to rest, they will annihilate with an electron normally into two photons, which are emitted in opposite directions. Both photons have energies of 511 keV in the center-of-mass system, corresponding to the rest mass of the annihilated positron and electron.

2.2.1 Energy loss of electrons/positrons

The energy loss of electrons in the matter can be calculated with the Bethe-Bloch formula, which needs modification, is described by[1]

$$-\left\langle \frac{dE}{dx} \right\rangle_{Ionization} \propto \ln(E) \tag{7}$$

---

[1] The exact ionization energy loss of electrons for z = 1, is given by $-\frac{dE}{dx} = 4\pi N_A r_e^2 m_e c^2 \frac{Z}{A}\frac{1}{\beta^2}\left[\ln\left(\frac{\gamma m_e c^2}{2I}\right) - \beta^2 - \frac{\delta^*}{2}\right]$, the parameter δ^* takes different values of the δ for the heavy charged particles.

Dominating process for $E_e > 10–30$ MeV is not anymore ionization but the effect of Bremsstrahlung, where an electron accelerated in the Coulomb field of nucleus produces photon emission

$$-\left\langle \frac{dE}{dx} \right\rangle_{Brem} \propto \frac{E}{m^2} \tag{8}$$

usually the energy loss due to Bremsstrahlung is written:

$$-\left\langle \frac{dE}{dx} \right\rangle_{Brem} \propto \frac{E}{X_0}, \quad X_0 = \frac{A}{4aN_A Z^2 r_e^2 \ln \frac{183}{Z^{1/3}}} \tag{9}$$

X_0 = radiation length in [g/cm^2].

The physical property of the radiation length for a material is that after passage of one X_0, the electron has lost all but $(1/e)^{th}$ of its initial energy [9]

It is also defined a critical energy E_c, for which the energy loss due to ionization is equivalent to energy loss due to Bremsstrahlung:

$$\left. \frac{dE}{dx}(E_c) \right|_{Brems} = \left. \frac{dE}{dx}(E_c) \right|_{Ion} \tag{10}$$

In **Figure 3**, the electron energy loss is presented in Copper. The critical energy in this case is about 25 MeV.

2.2.2 Range of electrons/positrons

The range of low-energy electrons (0.5 MeV ≤ Ekin ≤5 MeV) in Aluminum is described [10] by

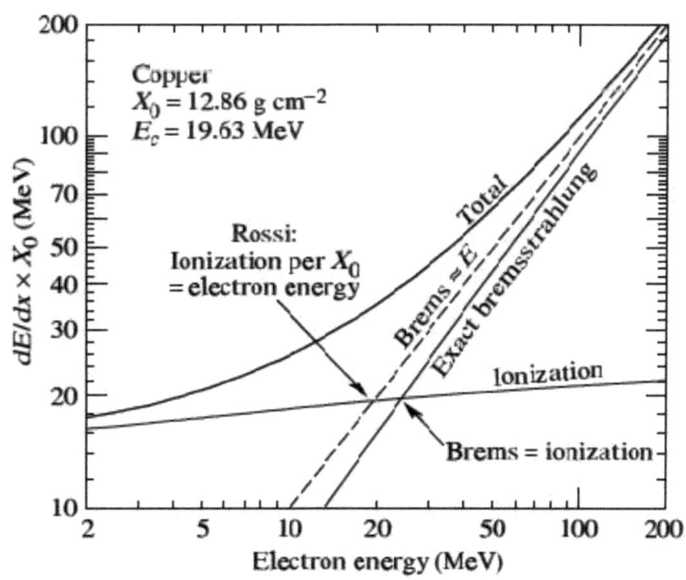

Figure 3.
The electron energy loss is shown under the ionization and the Bremsstrahlung effect for an energy range 2–200 MeV.

$$R_e = 0.526\left(E_{kin}/MeV - 0.094\right)g/cm^2 \quad (11)$$

In **Figure 5** the electron range is plotted for various energies of electrons penetrating through a certain Aluminum absorber thickness [10, 11]. This figure shows the difficulty in the definition of a range of a particle due to the pronounced range straggling, in this case mainly due to the fact that electrons will experience multiple scattering and bremsstrahlung in the absorber. The extrapolation of the linear part of the curves shown in **Figure 4** to the intersection with the abscissa defines the practical range [11].

2.3 Linear energy transfer

The term "linear energy transfer (LET)" is used to indicate the average amount of energy that is lost per unit path-length as a charged particle travels through a given material and deposited in it. The LET for electrons is traditionally expressed in units of MeV/cm. In case, the value is divided by the mass density, then in units of MeV-cm^2/g. The average amount of energy deposited in a thin sample, per electron, can be estimated by multiplying the LET by the sample thickness. Similarly, the total energy deposited per gram of a specimen, following an exposure of N electrons/area, is

$$E = \frac{LET \cdot N}{\rho} \quad (12)$$

where, ρ is the mass density of the specimen material.

The energy deposited per gram is referred to as the radiation dose. Radiation doses are usually expressed in rads in the older literature, where 1 rad is equal to 100 erg/g. Alternatively the dose is expressed in the Standard International (SI) units of gray (Gy), where 1Gy = 1 J/kg, and thus 1 rad = 0.01 Gy. Since the dose is proportional to the electron exposure, it is commonly used to refer to the exposure as being the "dose." While this terminology is not strictly correct, the intended meaning becomes understandable in context.

2.4 Interaction of photons: attenuation

Photons are detected indirectly via interactions in the material passed through. Subsequent ionization in the matter provides charged particles, which are spread

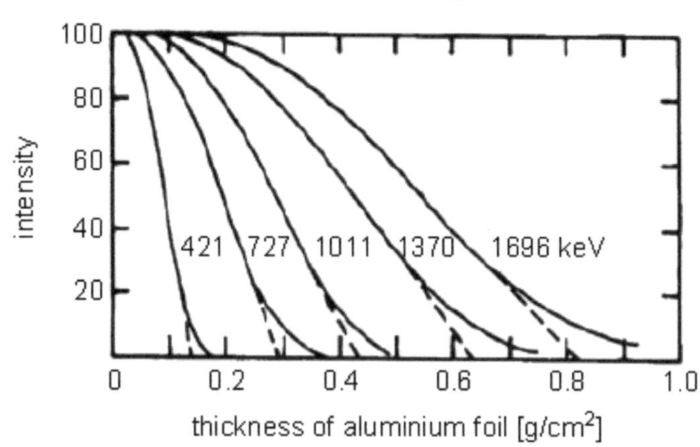

Figure 4.
Absorption of electrons of various energies in aluminum foils [10, 11].

through. Interactions of photons are fundamentally different from ionization processes of charged particles because in every photon interaction, the photon is either completely absorbed (photoelectric effect, pair production) or scattered through a relatively large angle meaning the Compton effect. Since the absorption or scattering is a statistical process, it is impossible to define a range for γ rays. A photon beam is attenuated exponentially in matter according to.

$$I = I_0 e^{-\mu x} \tag{13}$$

The length x in Eq. (13) is an area density with the unit g/cm^2. If the length is measured in cm, the mass attenuation coefficient μ must be divided by the density ρ of the material. The mass attenuation coefficient μ is related to the cross sections for the various interaction processes of photons according to

$$\mu = \frac{N_A}{A} \sum_i \sigma_i \tag{14}$$

where σ_i is the atomic cross section for the process i, A is the atomic weight and N_A is the Avogadro number. The mass attenuation coefficient, according to Eq. (14) given per g/cm^2, depends strongly on the photon energy.

2.4.1 Photoelectric effect

Atomic electrons absorb the energy of a photon completely. This effect is not possible for free electrons due to momentum conservation. The absorption of a photon by an atomic electron requires a third collision partner, which in this case is the atomic nucleus. The cross section for absorption of a photon of energy E_γ in the K shell is extremely large (≈80% of the total cross section), because of the proximity of the third collision partner, the atomic nucleus, which absorbs the recoil momentum. The total photoelectric cross section in the non-relativistic range away from the absorption edges is given in the non-relativistic Born approximation by [12]

$$\sigma^K_{photo} = \left(\frac{32}{\varepsilon^7}\right)^{1/2} \alpha^4 \cdot Z^5 \cdot \sigma^e_{Th} \left[cm^2/atom\right] \tag{15}$$

where, $\varepsilon = E_\gamma / m_e c^2$ is the reduced photon energy and

$$\sigma^e_{Th} = \frac{8}{3}\pi r_e^2 = 6.65 \cdot 10^{-25}\, cm^2 \tag{16}$$

is the Thomson cross section for elastic scattering of photons on electrons.

For higher energies (ε >> 1) the energy dependence of the cross section for the photoelectric effect is much less pronounced,

$$\sigma^K_{photo} = 4\pi r_e^2 \alpha^4 \cdot Z^5 \cdot \frac{1}{\varepsilon} \tag{17}$$

In Eqs. (15) and (17) the Z dependence of the cross section is approximated by Z^5. This indicates that the photon does not interact with an isolated atomic electron. Z-dependent corrections, however, cause σ_{photo} to be a more complicated function of Z. In the energy range between 0.1 MeV ≤ Eγ ≤ 5 MeV the exponent of Z varies between 4 and 5. As a consequence of the photoelectric effect in an inner shell (e.g., of the K shell) secondary effects may occur, as the free place, e.g., in the K shell, is filled by an electron from a higher shell, the energy difference between those two shells can be liberated in the form of X rays of characteristic energy.

2.4.1.1 Compton scattering

The Compton effect is the scattering of photons off quasi-free atomic electrons. In the study of this interaction process, the binding energy of the atomic electrons is neglected. The total cross section for Compton scattering per electron is given by [12]

$$\sigma_c^e = 2\pi r_e^2 \left\{ \left(\frac{1+\varepsilon}{\varepsilon}\right)\left[\frac{2(1+\varepsilon)}{1+2\varepsilon} - \frac{1}{\varepsilon}\ln(1+2\varepsilon)\right] + \frac{1}{2\varepsilon}\ln(1+2\varepsilon) - \frac{1+3\varepsilon}{(1+2\varepsilon)^2} \right\}\left[cm^2/electron\right], \quad \varepsilon = \frac{E_\gamma}{m_e c^2} \quad (18)$$

For Compton scattering off atoms the cross section is increased by the factor Z, because there are exactly Z electrons as possible scattering centers in an atom; consequently $\sigma_c^{atomic} = Z \cdot \sigma_c^e$.

In Compton-scattering process only a fraction of the photon energy is transferred to the electron. Therefore, one defines an energy scattering cross section

$$\sigma_{cs} = \frac{E'_\gamma}{E_\gamma} \cdot \sigma_c^e \quad (19)$$

where, the energy $E'_\gamma = E_\gamma - E_{kin}$ and the E_{kin} is transferred to the target electron.

The Compton scattering is a special effect for photon interactions, because only part of the photon energy is transferred to the target electron, one has to distinguish between the mass attenuation coefficient and the mass absorption coefficient. The mass attenuation coefficient μ_{cs} is related to the Compton-energy scattering cross section σ_{cs}, as in Eq. (19), according to Eq. (14). Correspondingly, the mass absorption coefficient μ_{ca} is calculated from the energy absorption cross-section σ_{ca}, Eq. (14). For various absorbers the Compton-scattering cross sections, or absorption coefficients, have been multiplied by the atomic number of the absorber, since the Compton scattering cross section, Eq. (18), given by the Klein–Nishina formula is valid per electron, but in this case, the atomic cross sections are required.

2.4.2 Pair production

The production of electron–positron pairs in the Coulomb field of a nucleus is only possible if the photon energy exceeds a certain threshold. This threshold energy is given by the rest masses of two electrons plus the recoil energy, which is transferred to the nucleus. From energy and momentum conservation, this threshold energy can be calculated to be

$$E_\gamma \geq 2m_e c^2 + 2\frac{m_e^2}{m_{nucleus}} c^2 \quad (20)$$

but usually $m_{nucleus} \gg m_e$ the effective threshold can be approximately

$$E_\gamma \geq 2m_e c^2 \quad (21)$$

The pair-production cross section is given by [22]

$$\sigma_{pair} = 4\alpha r_e^2 \cdot Z^2 \left(\frac{7}{9} \ln 2\varepsilon - \frac{109}{54} \right) \left[cm^2/atom \right] \tag{22}$$

For large photon energies, the pair-production cross section approaches an energy-independent value which is given approximately by

$$\sigma_{pair} \approx \frac{7}{9} 4\alpha r_e^2 \cdot Z^2 \ln \frac{183}{Z^{1/3}} \approx \frac{7}{9} \cdot \frac{A}{N_A} \cdot \frac{1}{X_0} \tag{23}$$

2.4.3 Total photon absorption cross section and mass attenuation coefficient

Ranges, in which the individual photon interaction processes dominate, are plotted in **Figure 5** as a function of the photon energy and the atomic number of the absorber [11, 12].

The total mass attenuation coefficient, which is related to the cross sections according to Eq. (14), is shown in **Figures 6–9** for the absorbers water, air, Aluminum and Lead [13, 14].

The μ_{ph} is the absorption coefficient for the photoelectric effect, μ_{cs} the Compton scattering, μ_{ca} the Compton absorption and μ_p the pair production. So μ_a is the total mass absorption coefficient ($\mu_a = \mu_{ph} + \mu_p + \mu_{ca}$).

Further interactions of photons (photonuclear interactions, photon–photon scattering, etc.) are governed by extremely low cross sections.

Therefore, these processes are of little importance for the detection of photons. However, these processes are of large interest in elementary particle physics and particle astrophysics.

2.5 Radiation detection

The detection of ionizing radiation in various energy ranges from keV to MeV is presented. The physical processes of radiation/matter interaction have been introduced in the previous text. All the steps of detection are covered, as well as detectors, instrumentations and measurements methods commonly used in the

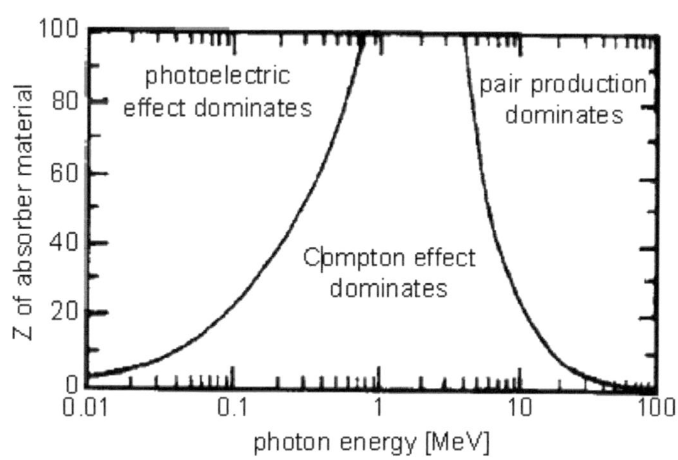

Figure 5.
Ranges in which the photoelectric effect, Compton effect and pair production dominate as a function of the photon energy and the target charge number Z [11, 12].

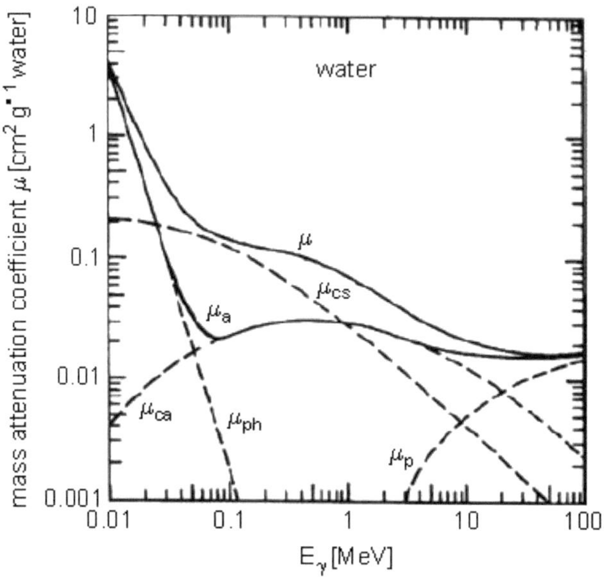

Figure 6.
Energy dependence of the mass attenuation coefficient μ and mass absorption coefficient μ_a for photons in water.

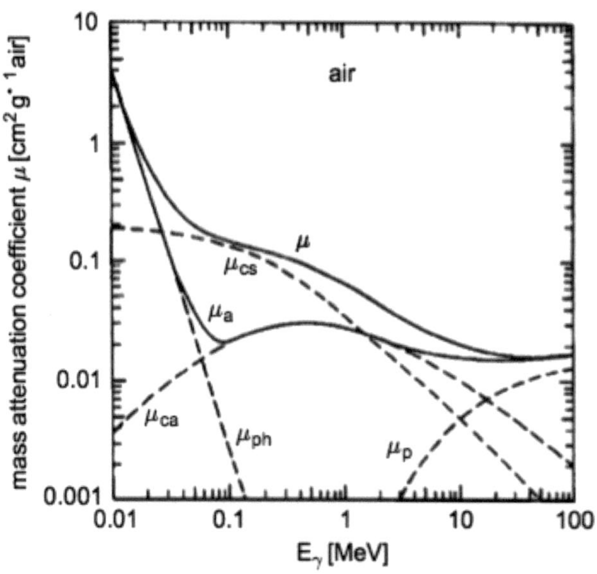

Figure 7.
Energy dependence of the mass attenuation coefficient μ and mass absorption coefficient μ_a for photons in Air.

nuclear field. There are many radiation detectors being developed so far. A selection of the most characteristic detectors will be presented, having played crucial role to the nuclear imaging.

2.5.1 Ionizing chambers

This radiation detector is based on the effects produced by a charged particle passing through a gas. The primary modes of interaction involve ionization and

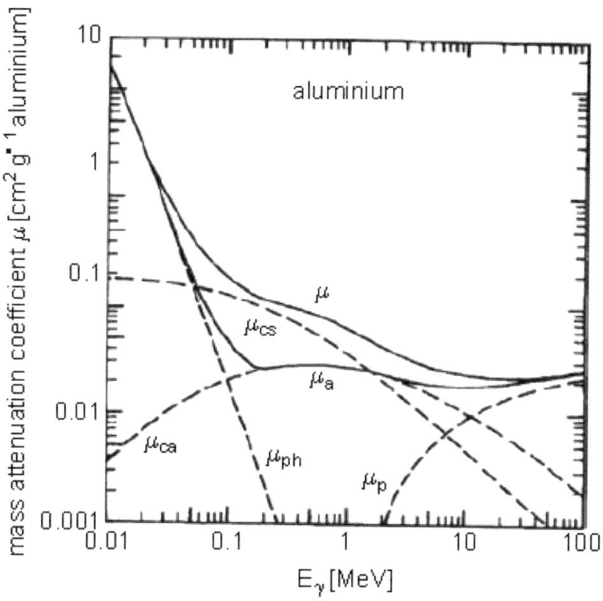

Figure 8.
Energy dependence of the mass attenuation coefficient μ and mass absorption coefficient μ_a for photons in Aluminum.

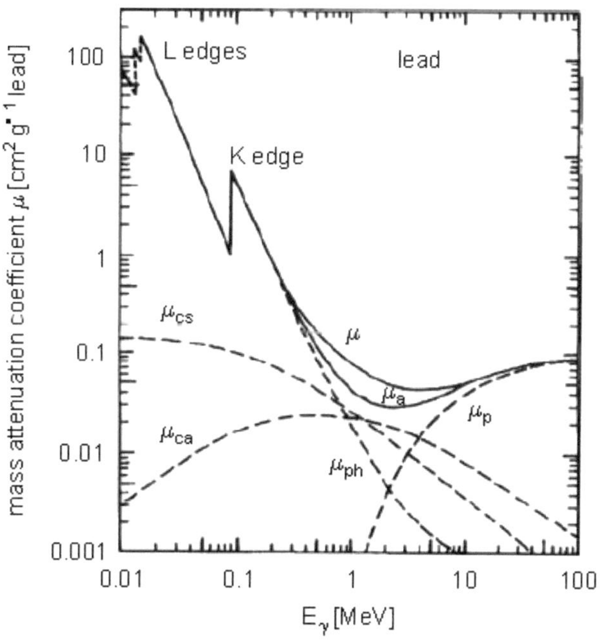

Figure 9.
Energy dependence of the mass attenuation coefficient μ and mass absorption coefficient μ_a for photons in Lead.

excitation of gas molecules along the particle track. An electronic output signal is derived originating from the ion pairs formed within the gas filling the detector. The charged particle transfers an amount of energy equal to the ionization energy of the gas molecule to permit the ionization process to occur. In most gases of interest for radiation detectors, the ionization energy for the least tightly bound electron shells is roughly 10 to 25 eV. The neutral atoms or molecules of the gas are in constant thermal motion; characterized by a mean free path for typical gases under standard conditions of about 10^6–10^8 m. A typical value of the average energy lost by the incident particle per ion pair formed is 25–35 eV/ion pair. Therefore, an incident 1 MeV particle, if it is fully stopped within the gas, will create about 30,000 ion pairs. A point-like collection of free electrons spread around the original point into a Gaussian spatial distribution; where the width increases by the time. An external electric field is applied to the ionization chamber; where ions or electrons created in the gas by the incident particle, electrostatic forces tend to move the charges away from their point of origin. The net motion consists of a superposition of a random thermal velocity together with a net drift velocity in a given direction. The drift velocity for positive ions is in the direction of the conventional electric field, whereas free electrons and negative ions drift in the opposite direction. Finally the total charge collection constitutes an electric current, the called ionization current. The magnitude of the ionization current is too small to be measured usually by a galvanometer. An active amplification of the current is implemented by sensing the voltage drop across a series resistance placed in the measuring circuit. The voltage developed across the resistor (i.e., a value of 10^9–10^{12} Ohms) can be amplified used for the measured signal. An alternative approach is to convert the signal from dc to ac at an early stage, which then allows a more stable amplification of the ac signal in subsequent stages. This conversion is accomplished in the dynamic-capacitor or vibrating reed electrometer by collecting the ion current across an RC circuit with long time constant. A charge Q is stored on the capacitance, which is given by Q = CV. If a charge ΔQ is created by the radiation, then the total charge stored on the capacitance will be reduced by ΔQ. The voltage will therefore drop from its original value of V_o by an amount ΔV given by.

$$\Delta V = \frac{\Delta Q}{C} \tag{24}$$

A measurement of ΔV provides the total ionization charge or the integrated ionization current over the period of the measurement.

2.5.2 Scintillator detectors

Scintillation detectors offer one possibility of providing a solid detection medium, and their application to the detection and measurement of various radiations. The detection of ionizing radiation by the scintillation light produced in certain materials is a very well established technique and remains one of the most useful methods available for the detection and spectroscopy of a wide variety of radiations. The kinetic energy of charged particles is converted into detectable light, by subsequent photosensitive detector, with high scintillation process efficiency. The conversion is taken care to be linear and the light yield to be proportional to the deposited energy over the most possible wide range. The scintillating material should be transparent to the wavelength of its own emission for total light collection. The decay time of the induced luminescence is short and then fast signal pulses can be generated. The process of fluorescence is the prompt emission of visible radiation from a substance following its excitation by incident radiation. It is conventional to distinguish several other processes that can also lead to the emission of visible light. The scintillation efficiency of any scintillator is defined as the fraction of all incident particle energy, which is converted into visible light. The rise and fall of the light output can be characterized by the full width at half maximum (FWHM) of the resulting light versus time profile, which can be measured using very fast timing procedures. It has become common to specify the performance of ultrafast organic scintillators by their FWHM time rather than the decay time alone. It is noted that both rise and decay time are of the order of ns. The alkali halide scintillators as the Sodium Iodide with trace of Thallium NaI(Tl) and the Cesium Iodide with trace of Thallium or Sodium CsI(Tl)/CsI(Na) are so broadly implemented for gamma spectroscopy and medical imaging applications. An alternative scintillation material, $Bi_4Ge_3O_{12}$ (BGO) is available as crystals of reasonable size. A major advantage is the high density (7.13 g/cm^3) and the large atomic number (83) of the Bismuth element. These properties result in the largest probability per unit volume for the photoelectric absorption of gamma rays. Its physical properties make it easy to handle and use. The light yield from BGO is relatively low, being variously reported at 10–20% of that of NaI(Tl).

2.5.3 Si/Ge solid state detectors

The use of a solid detection medium in many radiation detection applications is of great advantage, as for the measurement of high-energy electrons or gamma rays. The detector dimensions can be kept much smaller than the equivalent gas-filled detector because the solid densities are some 1000 times greater than that for a gas. The use of semiconductor materials as radiation detectors can result in a much larger number of carriers for a given incident radiation event than is possible with any other common detector type, described previously. Consequently, the best energy resolution from radiation spectrometers is achieved using semiconductor detectors. The fundamental information carriers are electron-hole pairs created along the path taken by the charged particle of the primary radiation or secondary particle through the detector. The electron-hole pair is somewhat analogous to the ion pair created in gas-filled detectors. Their motion in an applied electric field generates the basic electrical signal from the detector. Under low values of the electric field intensity, the drift velocity v is proportional to the applied field. Then a mobility μ for both electrons and holes can be defined by.

$$v_e = \mu_e E \quad v_h = \mu_h E \tag{25}$$

where, E is the electric field magnitude. We have seen, that the mobility of the free electron in the gas is much larger than of the positive ion, but in semiconductor materials the mobility of the electron and hole are roughly of the same order, saturated by the increased electric field to value of the order of 10^7 cm/s. When a charged particle passes through a semiconductor the overall significant effect is the production of many equal numbers electron–hole pairs along the track of the particle. The process produces high-energy electrons or delta rays that subsequently lose their energy in producing more electron–hole pairs. This quantity, is called the ionization energy, is experimentally observed to be largely independent of both the energy and type of the incident radiation, provided the charge particle is fully stopped within the active volume of the detector.

The Si surface barrier detectors have widespread application for the detection of alpha particles and other short-range radiations but are not easily adaptable for applications that involve more penetrating radiations. Their major limitation is the maximum depletion depth or active volume that can be created. Using Silicon or Germanium of normal semiconductor purity, depletion depths beyond 2 or 3 mm are difficult to achieve despite applying bias voltages that are near the breakdown level. A low impurity concentration corresponds to levels that are less than 1 part in 1012, a virtually unprecedented degree of material purity. Techniques have been developed to achieve this goal in Germanium, but not in Silicon. The process of Lithium ion drifting has been applied in both Silicon, Si(Li), and Germanium, Ge (Li), crystals to compensate the material after the crystal has been grown. Detectors that are manufactured from this ultrapure Germanium are usually called high purity Germanium (HPGe) detectors, and they have become available with depletion depths of several centimeters. The room-temperature operation of Germanium detectors is impossible because of the large thermally induced leakage current, due to the small band gap (~1 eV). So, the Germanium detectors must be cooled to reduce the leakage current to the point that the associated noise does not spoil their excellent energy resolution. Normally, the operation temperature is at 77 K through the use of an insulated Dewar vessel, which a reservoir of liquid Nitrogen is kept in thermal contact with the detector. For Ge(Li) detectors, the low temperature must be maintained continuously to prevent a catastrophic redistribution of the drifted lithium that will rapidly take place at room temperature.

2.5.4 Pixel detectors

The approach to obtain two-dimensional position information from a single sided silicon detector is to fabricate the top electrode as a checkerboard pattern of individual small elements that are electrically isolated from each other. If the electrode dimensions are smaller than 1 mm, the common terminology is pixel detector. Electrical connection must be made to each individual electrode and separate electronic readout channels provided for each. This approach has the advantage that the small size of each individual electrode results in a relatively small capacitance and leakage current, and thus the electronic noise is reduced considerably from that observed from microstrip detectors of equivalent dimensions. In the usual approach, a pixel detector chip is connected to a separate readout chip using flip chip solder bonding or Indium bump bonds. The readout chip is fabricated with exactly the same pitch as the detector pixels, so each bump provides an electrical connection between a single pixel and its corresponding readout electronics. Pixel detectors typically have active areas that are limited to the order of square centimeters. Larger detector areas can be achieved by assembling individual modules into arrays, although at the expense of increasing complexity in what is already a complex device.

2.6 Electronics and DAQ

Complicated electronic systems are adapted to get the information of the signal extraction by the radiation detectors. After an analog and digital treatment of the detector plus electronics waveform; a data acquisition system (DAQ) is accumulating the data for further analysis and study.

2.6.1 Signal processing and analysis: types of electronics, signal collection and amplification, particle discrimination, spatial and time resolution

It is often desirable to change the shape of the pulse signal from radiation detectors, in some predetermined fashion. It is the most common application in processing a train of pulses produced by a preamplifier. In order to ensure that complete charge collection occurs, preamplifiers are normally adjusted to provide a decay time for the pulse, which is quite long, typically 50 μs. Depending of the rate of interaction in the detector these pulses will tend to overlap one another and give rise to a pulse train. The ideal shape is to eliminate the long tails of the pulses, but the information carried by the maximum amplitude of the pulse has been preserved. The pulses have been shaped in the sense that their total length has been reduced drastically but not affecting the maximum amplitude. The nuclear pulse shaping, it is conventional to make an important distinction between differentiator or CR networks and integrator or RC. Both operations can also be thought of as filtering in the frequency domain, for pulse shaping to improve signal-to-noise ratio by limiting the response of the instrumentation to those frequency ranges in which the signal has useful components. This type of pulse shaping is conventionally carried out in the linear amplifier element of a nuclear pulse signal chain and then to the digital pulse processing, for getting a digitized version of the input waveform for further analysis. A linear pulse is defined as a signal pulse that carries information through its amplitude, and sometimes by its shape as well. A sequence of linear pulses may therefore differ widely in size and shape characteristics. In addition, a logic pulse is a signal pulse of standard size and shape that carries information only by its presence or absence, or by the precise time of its appearance. Usually, all radiation detector signal chains start out with linear pulses, which after passing fixed amplitude discrimination, a digital conversion provides the logic pulses by the ADC (Analog to Digital Converter) elements. The information on the precise arrival time of a quantum of radiation in the detector is of particular interest. The accuracy of the timing information to be performed depends both on the properties of the specific detector, where the signal charge is collected rapidly and the type of electronics used to process the signal. The timing characteristics of a certain system depend greatly on the dynamic range, ratio of maximum to minimum pulse height, of the signal pulses. The time resolution is defined by the time measurement accuracy of the system. Similar spatial resolution of a nuclear chain is defined for acquiring the discrimination of two same radiation quanta passing in nearby places of a detector.

2.6.2 Multi-channel analysis and measurements: principle of measurements, spectrometry, common detection instrumentations, applications in nuclear engineering and R&D

A measurement of the differential pulse height spectrum from a radiation detector can yield important information on the nature of the incident radiation or the properties of the detector itself and is therefore one of the most important functions to be performed in nuclear measurements. By definition, the differential pulse height spectrum is a continuous curve that plots the value of dN/dH, the differential number of pulses observed within a differential increment of pulse height H, versus the value of the pulse height H.

The multichannel analyzer (MCA) is comprised of basic electronics components chain setup. The major task of its operation is based on the principle of converting an analog signal (the pulse amplitude) to an equivalent digital number. Then, an extensive technology available for the storage and display of the digital information provides the recording pulse height spectra. As a result, the analog to-digital converter (ADC) is a key element in determining the performance characteristics of the analyzer.

The nuclear instrumentation, mainly, based by the detector, the electronic system, the MCA and the data storage-analysis medium, can be properly adapted for several applications. Those applications are starting form the nuclear engineering instrumentation for nuclear reactors monitoring and safety, to various research instrumentations for accelerators or detector systems and so on. All these experience of the nuclear instrumentation, accumulated the last decades, is implemented to the medical applications and indeed to the nuclear medical imaging techniques.

3. The X-ray computed tomography imaging

The X-rays are high-energy photons produced via special vacuum tubes. The X-rays are proportionally attenuated when passing through various media; being the major advantage for the X-ray imaging. The updated medical diagnosis result of this technology is the three-dimensional (3D) X-ray computed tomography (CT), used in medical diagnosis.

3.1 X-ray generation and interaction with matter

A typical X-ray tube consists of a cathode providing, by thermal emission, beam of electrons accelerated due to the anode voltage. Kinetic energy loss of the electrons at an anode is converted to X-rays. The relative position of the excited electron in the anode determines the frequency and energy of the emitted X-ray. The X-rays interact with matter in several ways, as the photon interaction mechanisms, reported in paragrap. 1.4; meaning the Photoelectric effect, Compton scattering and Pair production. The major effect in diagnostic imaging is the photoelectric effect; where an orbital electron, mainly for elements of large atomic number, absorbs the energy of an X-ray photon.

3.2 CT imaging

The established X-ray imaging technique is useful for clinical diagnosis in cases of a view of the bone system. The technique offers only low soft-tissue contrast and is not very quantitative. The X-ray CT tomography relies on taking a large number of X-rays at multiple angles, getting many measurements of the incident X-ray attenuation through the plane of the human body. The attenuation measurements provide the fraction of X-ray removed in passing through a given amount of a specific material of thickness. The data obtained provide the X-ray tomography information and reconstruct a 3D image after a heavy and well elaborated data processing. The computed tomography (CT) is the method for reconstructing and providing the image of a thin cross section on the basis of measurements of X-ray attenuation. Instead, the plain film X-ray image, CT images are free of superimposing tissues and are capable of much higher contrast due to elimination of scatter. Major upgrading improvements have led to higher-resolution images, which the diagnosis process. The small size nodules or tumors can be visualized, by the CT scan, which they could not be seen with a plain X-ray film. To help soft tissues providing clear image, a special contrast material is needed to block the X-rays, in a CT scan, so highlighting blood vessels, organs, or other structures.

4. The nuclear medicine SPECT, PET and PET-CT tomography imaging

Nuclear medicine is a branch of medical imaging applying non-invasive, diagnostic imaging techniques for visualization of internal organs, tissue, etc. and monitoring the functioning of them. Major modalities of imaging are the X-ray Radiography (projection), the X-ray Computed Tomography (CT) and the Nuclear Medicine (SPECT, PET and PET-CT) [15, 16]. The injected radioactive tracers (radiopharmaceuticals) to human body assess tissue functions and to diagnose and treat properly various diseases but mainly malignant tissues. Specially designed cameras track the path of these radioactive tracers. Single Photon Emission Computed Tomography or SPECT and Positron Emission Tomography or PET scans are the two most common imaging modalities in nuclear medicine. The PET-CT scan is a combination of the PET and the CT-computed tomography, described above, which give excellent results of the cancer spots inside the body not viewed via PET or CT separately. Approved tracers are called radiopharmaceuticals since they must meet FDA's[2] or EMA's[3] exacting standards for safety and appropriate performance for the approved clinical use. The proper tracer is selected to provide the most specific and reliable information for a patient's particular problem. The used tracer is determined by the SPECT or PET scan to be applied to the patient [17].

4.1 SPECT imaging

The SPECT imaging scanner provides three-dimensional tomographic images of the distribution of radioactive tracer molecules that have been introduced into the patient's body. The 3D images are computer generated from a large number of projection images of the body recorded at different angles. The SPECT imagers have gamma camera detectors that can detect the gamma ray emissions from the tracers that have been injected into the patient [18]. The camera sensor detectors are mounted on a rotating gantry that allows them to be moved in a tight circle around a patient who is lying motionless on a moving bed [19]. The SPECT scans are primarily used to diagnose and track the progression of heart disease, such as blocked coronary arteries. There are also radiotracers to detect disorders in bone, gall bladder disease and intestinal tuberculosis or bleeding. The SPECT agents have recently become available for aiding in the diagnosis of Parkinson's disease in the brain, and distinguishing this disease from other anatomically related movement disorders and dementias [20]. The gamma camera has usually a set of photomultipliers on a scintillating crystal in front of which the collimator defines the image quality to be obtained, **Figure 10**. The collimator localizing the origin of the gamma ray forms a projection image by allowing only those gamma rays traveling in certain directions to reach the scintillating crystal.

4.2 PET imaging

The PET scan also uses special radiopharmaceuticals to create three-dimensional images. These radiopharmaceuticals are labeled with radioisotopes (^{11}C, ^{18}F, ^{15}O or ^{13}N) of very short life-time (~minutes to few hours) and they emit positrons by their decay. The positrons are anti-particles of the electrons having positive charge. The positrons with electrons annihilate each other, in the human tissue where have been injected, emitting two gamma rays of equal energy 512 keV each in opposite directions due to the conservation of energy and momentum [20, 21]. The detectors in the PET scanner facility measure these photons emitted in time coincidence and in 180° angle. The PET camera also allows determining where they two photons are coming from, the position of the nucleus when it decayed, and also knowing where the nucleus moves inside the body. The data of the detectors obtained are processed for providing the information to create images of internal organs or tissues.

---

[2] FDA: U.S. FOOD & DRUG ADMINISTRATION, https://www.fda.gov/MedicalDevices/NewsEvents/WorkshopsConferences/ucm429282.htm

[3] EMA: EUROPEAN MEDICINES AGENCY, https://www.ema.europa.eu/

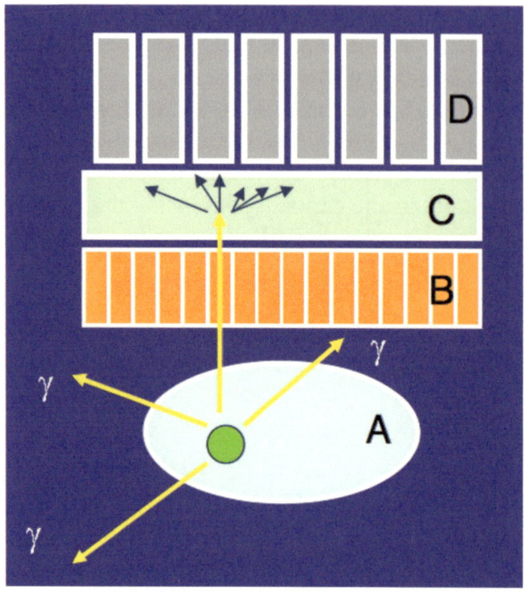

Figure 10.
The gamma camera setup (principle), A is the organ, and under examination, with the radiopharmaceutical compound emitting gamma rays, B is the collimator, C is the scintillating crystal and D is the array of the photomultipliers.

The PET scan is manly used for the patients with conditions affecting the brain, heart, certain types of cancer, Alzheimer's disease and some neurological disorders. The major purpose of PET scans is to detect cancer and monitor its progression, response to treatment, and to detect metastases. Glucose utilization depends on the intensity of cellular and tissue activity so it is greatly increased in rapidly dividing cancer cells. In the last years, slightly modified radiolabeled glucose molecules (F-18 labeled deoxyglucose or FDG) have been shown to be the best available tracer for detecting cancer and its metastatic spread in the body. Different colors or degrees of brightness on a PET image represent different levels of tissue or organ function. The healthy tissues use glucose for energy, accumulating some of the tagged glucose, which will show up on the PET images. However, the tumors use more glucose than normal tissue, accumulate more of the substance and appear brighter than normal tissue on the PET images.

4.3 PET-CT imaging

A combination instrument that produces both PET and CT scans of the same body regions in one examination (PET/CT scanner) has become the primary imaging tool for the staging of most cancers worldwide. The images of the PET and the PET-CT combined are shown in **Figure 11** [22]; where the results of the PET-CT image are extremely interesting. The incremental diagnostic value of integrated positron emission tomography-computed tomography (PET/CT) compared with PET tomography are summarized: (i) imaging quality improvement in tumors detection on both CT and PET, (ii) imaging quality improvement to the loci up taking tracer in better ratio between physiological from pathologic tissue, (iii) precise localization of the malignant foci, in various body places, i.e., bones, soft tissues, etc. (iv) improvement of spatial resolution for defining small size or unusual tumors. The use of PET/CT technique can occur at the time of initial diagnosis, in assessing the early response of disease to treatment, at the conclusion of treatment, and in continuing follow-up of patients. The PET/CT fused images

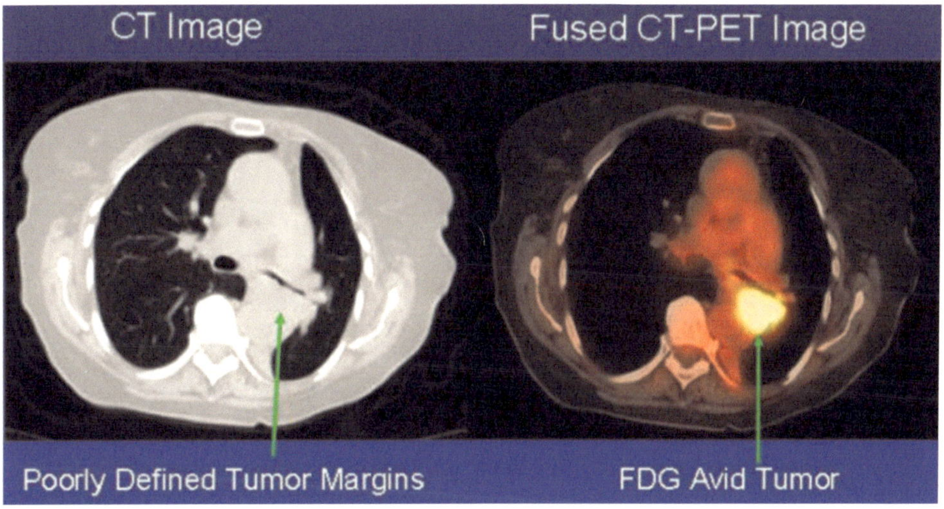

Figure 11.
The comparison between the CT image and the combined PET-CT image; where the avid tumor is well and clearly viewed on the right image (https://www.nibib.nih.gov/) [22].

have the potential to provide important information to guide the biopsy of a mass to active regions of the tumor and to provide better tissue mapping [22]. The wide array of clinical applications of ionizing radiation is grouped into diagnostic and therapeutic use [23].

The radiation dose and the diagnostic radiology procedures are of concern to the health care professions, the public, and regulators. The radiation dose depends on various factors, including the weight of the patient, the radiation sensitivity of the image tissue receptor, the energy of the radiation, the exposure rate, and the total time of radiation. Measurements of equivalent collective dose are taken for the individual patients and populations. The radiation dose from nuclear medicine procedures depends on the radiopharmaceutical, the administered activity, and individual patient metabolism. For clinical applications, dosimetry estimates of radiopharmaceuticals are provided based on standardized adult and child metabolic and anatomic models. Recently, the use of electron accelerators as radiation source equipped with an X-ray converter is increasing. However, gamma sources are difficult to replace, especially for use with non-uniform, high-density products [24]. Fourth generation of light sources are the X-ray free electron lasers (XFELs) [25]. They provide bright bursts of X-rays, where these pulses are both spatially coherent and ultra short in duration. New techniques have been developed, including diffract-before-destruction methods; where the short X-ray pulse scatters from the sample, providing the radiation-damage-free structures measurement. They have been applied to develop a technique called serial femtosecond crystallography (SFX), where a stream of tiny protein crystals is delivered into the focus of the XFEL [26]. The Crystal Clear is an international collaboration at CERN, active on research and development on inorganic scintillation materials for novel ionizing radiation detectors, for high-energy physics, better quality medical imaging (PET-SPECT) and industrial applications [27].

Author details

Evangelos Gazis
National Technical University of Athens, Athens, Greece

*Address all correspondence to: evangelos.gazis@cern.ch

References

[1] Enge H. Introduction to Nuclear Physics. Boston: Addison-Wesley; 1972

[2] Kleinknecht K. Detectors for Particle Radiation. Cambridge UK: Cambridge University Press; 1986

[3] William R. Leo, Techniques fro Nuclear and Particle Physics Experiments. 2nd ed. Berlin, Heidelberg, New York: Springer Verlag; 1994

[4] Knoll GF. Radiation Detection and Measurement. 3rd ed. New York: John Wiley & Sons; 1999

[5] Sitar B, Merson GI, Chechin VA, Budagov YA. Ionization Measurements in High Energy Physics. Springer Tracts in Modern Physics. Vol. 124. Berlin/Heidelberg: Springer; 1993

[6] Bethe HA. Theorie des Durchgangs schneller Korpuskularstrahlen durch Materie. Annalen der Physik. 1930;**5**:325-400

[7] Bloch F. Bremsvermogen von Atomen mit mehreren Elektronen. Zeitschrift für Physik. 1933;**81**:363-376

[8] Uehling EA. Penetration of heavy charged particles in matter. Annual Review of Nuclear and Particle Science. 1954;**4**:315-350

[9] Particle Data Group. Review of particle properties. Physical Review D. 2018;**98**:030001

[10] Marshall JS, Ward AG. Absorption curves and ranges for homogeneous β-rays. Canadian Journal of Research. 1937;**A15**:39-41

[11] Sauter E. Grundlagen des Strahlenschutzes. Berlin/München: Siemens AG; 1971. Grundlagen des Strahlenschutzes. Thiemig/München; 1982

[12] Marmier P, Sheldon E. Physics of Nuclei and Particles. Vol. 1. New York: Academic Press; 1969

[13] Evans RD. The Atomic Nucleus. New York: McGraw-Hill; 1955

[14] Grodstein GW. X-Ray attenuation coefficients from 10 keV to 100 MeV. National Bureau of Standards Supplement to Circular. 1957;**583**:1

[15] Hine GJ. Instrumentation in Nuclear Medicine. 1st ed. Cambridge MA: Academic Press; 1967

[16] Alazraki NP, Mishkin FS. Fundamentals of Nuclear Medicine. 2nd ed. New York: The Society of Nuclear Medicine; 1988

[17] Edward L. Alpen, Radiation Biophysics. 2nd Edition. San Diego CA: Academic Press; 1998

[18] Khoshakhlagh M et al. Development of scintillators in nuclear medicine. World Journal of Nuclear Medicine. 2015;**14**(3):156-159

[19] Fockler A, Voslar A, Guilbault J. Spatial resolution of gamma cameras for whole body bone imaging. Journal of Nuclear Medicine. 2016;**57** (Supplement 2):2828

[20] Webb A. Introduction to Biomedical Imaging. Hoboken NJ: John Wiley & Sons; 2003

[21] Hendee WR, Ritenour ER. Medical Imaging Physics. 4th Edition. New York: Wiley; 2002

[22] NIBIB-National Institute of Biomedical Imagine and Bioengineering Health & Human Services. Available from: https://www.nibib.nih.gov/science-education/science-topics/nuclear-medicine

[23] Gottfried K-LD, Penn G, editors. Radiation in Medicine, A Need For Regulatory Reform, Institute of Medicine (US) Committee for Review and Evaluation of the Medical Use Program of the Nuclear Regulatory Commission. Washington DC: National Academic Press; 1996

[24] Sun Y, Chmielewski AG. Chapter: Future developments in radiation processing. In: Applications of Ionizing Radiation in Materials Processing. 1st ed. Warszawa: Institute of Nuclear Chemistry and Technology; 2017

[25] Pellegrini C, Marinelli A, Reiche S. The physics of X-ray free-electron lasers. Reviews of Modern Physics. 2016;**88**:015006

[26] Martin-Garcia JM et al. Serial femtosecond crystallography: A revolution in structural biology. Archives of Biochemistry and Biophysics. 2016;**602**:32-47

[27] Medjoubi K et al. Performances and Applications of the CdTe- and Si-XPAD3 photon counting 2D detector. Journal of Instrumentation. 2011;**6**: C01080

Chapter 4

PET-CT Principles and Applications in Lung Cancer Management

Long Chen, Hua Sun and Yunchao Huang

Abstract

Lung cancer is the most common malignant cancer throughout the world; the positron emission tomography/computed tomography (PET-CT) combines both the metabolism information from PET and anatomy details from CT, which is the state of the art. This manuscript introduced the PET-CT and applications in lung cancer diagnosing, staging, and treatment. Several aspects including clinical features, classification, grading and pathology of the lung cancer, principles of PET-CT, and evaluation of diagnosing and treatment had been covered. Detailed demonstration of each cancer subtype, staging criteria, and classification was described. The content will benefit the clinical doctors as well as radiologists.

Keywords: lung cancer, PET-CT

1. Lung cancer: an overview

1.1 Clinical features

Totally lung cancer remains the first leading cause of cancer incidence and mortality, with about 2.1 million incidence and 1.8 million deaths in 2018 among 185 countries [1]. In 2018, an estimated 234,030 new cases of lung and bronchial cancer will be diagnosed, and 154,050 deaths are estimated to occur because of the disease [2]. The 5-year over survival rate is <20% once diagnosed [3]. Lung cancer is a unique disease for its etiologic agent is an addictive product cigarette, made and produced by an industry. Voluntary or involuntary (secondhand) cigarette smoking leads to nearly 90% cases, suggesting that effective public health policies to prevent initiation of smoking, oversight of tobacco products, and other tobacco control measures will play crucial roles in reducing lung cancer mortality [4]. Increased exposure to smoke from the burning of charcoal for heating and cooking is believed to contribute to the high lung cancer incidence, rather than smoking that is thought to be the leading cause of high lung cancer incidence in western countries [5].

1.2 Classification

1.2.1 Non-small cell lung cancer (NSCLC)

There are four major cell types of lung cancer according to the World Health Organization (WHO) classification: adenocarcinoma (ADC), squamous cell carcinoma (SCC), large cell carcinoma, and small cell carcinoma [6]. The first three types are also called non-small cell lung cancer, consisting of the most majority of all lung cancers. This molecular-based classification is important for therapeutic decision-making for several reasons: (i) overall survival was statistically superior for cisplatin/pemetrexed versus cisplatin/gemcitabine in patients with ADC (12.6 versus 10.9 months, respectively). In contrast, in SCC patients, there was a significant improvement in survival with cisplatin/gemcitabine versus cisplatin/pemetrexed (10.8 versus 9.4 months, respectively) [7]. (ii) SCC patients receiving treatment with carboplatin and paclitaxel plus bevacizumab (15 mg/kg) are prone to suffering from life-threatening major hemoptysis [8]. (iii) ADC patients are likely to harbor epidermal growth factor receptor (EGFR) mutations which are predictive of responsiveness to tyrosine kinase inhibitors (TKI).

Age, smoking history, previous cancer history, family history, occupational exposures, other lung diseases (chronic obstructive pulmonary disease [COPD], pulmonary fibrosis), exposure to infectious agents (e.g., endemic areas of fungal infections, tuberculosis) or risk factors, or history suggestive of infection are all potential or obvious risk factors.

1.2.2 Small cell lung cancer

Neuroendocrine tumors account for about 20% of lung cancers, and most are small cell lung cancer (SCLC) [9]. SCLC is sometimes called oat cell cancer, accounting for approximately 10–15% of lung cancers, and is considered as a separate entity from NSCLC due to its early metastases and relative response to chemotherapy and radiation. Unfortunately, although small cell lung cancer usually responds very well initially to treatment, long-term survival remains low. To be specific, the 5-year survival rate is 31% for stage I, 19% for stage II, 8% for stage IV, and only 2% for stage IV disease. There is no significant difference in the AJCC TNM staging system between NSCLC and SCLC. In fact, in addition to the TNM staging, SCLC can also be defined as "limited stage" when the tumor is encompassed within a tolerable radiation field or defined as "extensive stage" when the tumor is too large or too widespread to be encompassed within tolerable radiation field, according to the older Veterans Administration (VA) [10]. Then the NCCN Panel adopted a combined approach for staging SCLC using both the AJCC TNM staging system and the VA scheme for SCLC. In applying the TNM classifications to the VA system, the so-called limited-stage SCLC is defined as stage I to III (any T, any N, M0) which can be effectively treated with definitive radiation therapy, while extensive-stage SCLC is defined as stage IV (any T, any N, M1a/b) or T3-T4 harboring multiple lung nodules or having tumor volume that is too large to be encompassed in a tolerable radiation plan. Positron emission tomography-computed tomography (PET-CT) scan will be useful to assess for distant metastases when limited-stage disease is suspected, and a bone scan can be performed if PET-CT is ambiguous or not available; bone biopsy can be applied if the bone scan is equivocal. Although PET-CT is superior to PET or CT alone in detecting most metastatic sites, it is inferior to MR for the detection of brain metastases [11].

1.2.3 Rare carcinoma of the lung

Adenosquamous carcinoma (ASC) is a rare subtype of lung cancer, making up 0.4–4% of all lung cancer cases, and it is made up of two of the main tumor types: adenocarcinoma and squamous [12]. People suffering from ASC are prone to survive within a shorter time than those with pure lung adenocarcinomas or squamous cell carcinomas of the lung, no matter whether it is diagnosed earlier or later. In addition, the proportion of the adenocarcinoma/squamous cell component has no effect on the outcome. Cisplatin (a chemotherapy drug used in the squamous cancer cell) rather than the pemetrexed (commonly used in adenocarcinomas) tends to be more effective in the treatment of ASC. Some studies have shown that ASC has its own clinical characteristics: patients are mainly males, the average age is 68.7 years old, most patients with ASC have smoking history, and most of the diseases are located in the peripheral rather than the central segment [12].

Carcinoid tumors are a type of tumor that relates to the neuroendocrine system, accounting for about 1–6% of all lung tumors, and approximately a quarter of patients suffering from carcinoid have no symptoms at the time of discovery. Although a common X-ray or chest CT scan can detect this disease, ^{18}F-FDG PET-CT scans are not sensitive enough to discover it or see if they have spread distantly because no obvious uptake can be discovered. Consequently, octreotide rather than FDG will be given if some are suspected of having a carcinoid tumor [13].

Granular cell lung tumors are extremely rare, accounting for approximately 0.2% of all lung tumors. Narrowed airways, which are caused by small, firm, and solitary nodules, can always be found. However, in most situations, this kind of disease is benign. Malignant or cancerous granular cell lung is even rarer [14].

Sarcomatoid carcinomas are another rare lung carcinoma, making up 0.3–3% of all NSCLC. Some studies have shown that heavy smoking and exposure to asbestos possibly, at least partially, are responsible for this disease [15].

1.3 Molecular pathology of lung cancer

Traditionally, according to histological features, NSCLC has been classified into small cell and non-small cell lung cancers and further was subdivided into squamous cell carcinoma, adenocarcinoma, and large cell carcinoma. Historically, little attention was given to the differentiation of the specific subtypes because there are no therapeutic implications, especially prior to the 2004 WHO classification. Various driver mutations have been associated with these cancers over time [16]; the genetic alterations and specific protein expression level have attracted much attention (**Figure 1**).

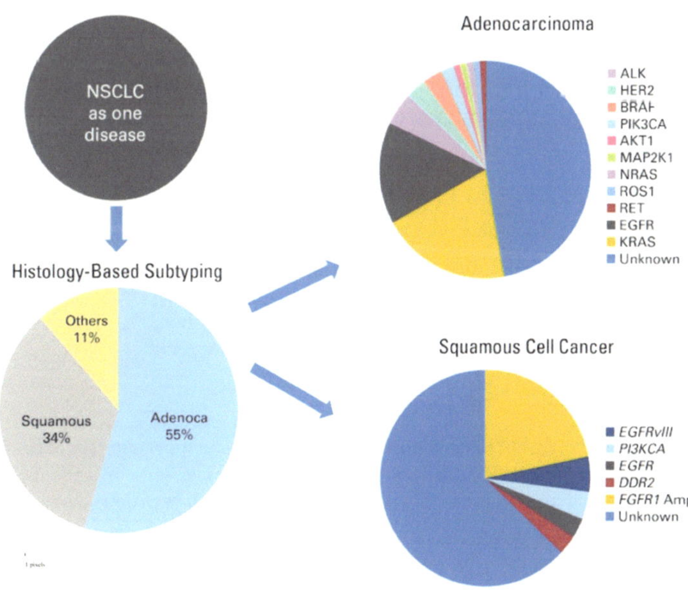

Figure 1.
Classifications of lung cancer: from histology to molecular based [16] (Reprinted with permission. © 2013 by the American Society of Clinical Oncology. All rights reserved).

1.4 TNM staging

The primary tumor (T), regional lymph node involvement (N), and distant metastasis (M) are the bases of staging for lung cancer. The International Association Society of Lung Cancer (IASLC) recommends the TNM classification of malignant tumors published by the Union Internationale Contre Le Cancer (UICC) and the American Joint Committee on Cancer (AJCC), and the latest eighth edition was published in 2016 [17]. Based on the different T, N, and M combinations, patients are grouped into different stages, which will determine the clinical treatments and can also predict various prognoses. The staging system is described in **Table 1**, and the stage groupings based on the TNM are listed in **Table 2**.

T—Primary tumor	
T category	T criteria
Tx	Primary tumor cannot be assessed, or tumor proven by the presence of malignant cells in sputum or bronchial washings but not visualized by imaging or bronchoscopy
T0	No evidence of primary tumor
Tis	Carcinoma in situ
	Squamous cell carcinoma in situ (SCIS)
	Adenocarcinoma in situ (AIS): adenocarcinoma with pure lepidic pattern, ≤3 cm in greatest dimension
T1	Tumor ≤3 cm in greatest dimension, surrounded by lung or visceral pleura, without bronchoscopic evidence of invasion more proximal than the lobar bronchus (i.e., not in the main bronchus)
T1mi	Minimally invasive adenocarcinoma: adenocarcinoma (≤3 cm in greatest dimension) with a predominantly lepidic pattern and ≤ 5 mm invasion in greatest dimension
T1a	Tumor ≤1 cm in greatest dimension. A superficial, spreading tumor of any size whose invasive component is limited to the bronchial wall and may extend proximal to the main bronchus; also is classified as T1a, but these tumors are uncommon
T1b	Tumor >1 cm but ≤2 cm in greatest dimension
T1c	Tumor >2 cm but ≤3 cm in greatest dimension
T2	Tumor >3 cm but ≤5 cm or having any of the following features: • Involves the main bronchus regardless of distance to the carina, but without involvement of the carina • Invades visceral pleura (PL1 or PL2) • Associated with atelectasis or obstructive pneumonitis that extends to the hilar region, involving part or all of the lung T2 tumors with these features are classified as T2a if ≤4 cm or if the size cannot be determined and T2b if >4 cm but ≤5 cm in greatest dimension
T2a	Tumor >3 cm but ≤4 cm in greatest dimension
T2b	Tumor >4 cm but ≤5 cm in greatest dimension
T3	Tumor >5 cm but ≤7 cm in greatest dimension or directly invading any of the following: parietal pleura (PL3), chest wall (including superior sulcus tumors), phrenic nerve, parietal pericardium; or separate tumor nodule (s) in the same lobe as the primary
T4	Tumor >7 cm or tumor of any size invading one or more of the following: the diaphragm, mediastinum, heart, great vessels, trachea, recurrent laryngeal nerve, esophagus, vertebral body, or carina; separate tumor nodule(s) in an ipsilateral lobe different from that of the primary
N—Regional lymph	
N category	N criteria

NX	Regional lymph nodes cannot be assessed
N0	No regional lymph node metastasis
N1	Metastasis in ipsilateral peribronchial and/or ipsilateral hilar lymph nodes and intrapulmonary nodes, including involvement by direct extension
N2	Metastasis in ipsilateral mediastinal and/or subcarinal lymph node(s)
N3	Metastasis in contralateral mediastinal, contralateral hilar, ipsilateral or contralateral scalene, or supraclavicular lymph node(s)
M category	M criteria
M0	No distant metastasis
M1	Distant metastasis
M1a	Separate tumor nodule(s) in a contralateral lobe; tumor with pleural or pericardial nodules or malignant pleural or pericardial effusion. Most pleural (pericardial) effusions with lung cancer are a result of the tumor. In a few patients, however, multiple microscopic examinations of pleural (pericardial) fluid are negative for tumor, and the fluid is nonbloody and not an exudate. If these elements and clinical judgment dictate that the effusion is not related to the tumor, the effusion should be excluded as a staging descriptor
M1b	Single extrathoracic metastasis in a single organ (including involvement of a single nonregional node)
M1c	Multiple extrathoracic metastases in a single organ or in multiple organs

Table 1.
The eighth edition of TNM for lung cancer.

Stage group	T	N	M
Stage IA	T1	N0	M0
Stage IA1	T1mi, T1a	N0	M0
Stage IA2	T1b	N0	M0
Stage IA3	T1c	N0	M0
Stage IB	T2a	N0	M0
Stage IIA	T2b	N0	M0
Stage IIB	T1a-c, T2a, b	N1	M0
	T3	N0	M0
Stage IIIA	T1a-c, T2a, b	N2	M0
	T3	N1	M0
	T4	N0, N1	M0
Stage IIIB	T1a-c, T2a, b	N3	M0
	T3, T4	N2	M0
Stage IIIC	T3, T4	N3	M0
Stage IVA	Any T	Any N	M1a, b
Stage IVB	Any T	Any N	M1c

Table 2.
Stage groupings in the eighth edition of TNM staging system for lung cancer.

1.5 Synoptic reporting of lung cancer

Synoptic reporting for lung cancer aimed to standardize diagnostic reports, including recommended clinical and histopathologic variables. This includes the

Terms
Clinical details
Clinical information provided on request Nature of the resection Additional extrapulmonary tissue Site and laterality of tumor Results of previous cytological investigations or biopsies Details of any previous treatment of the current tumor Details of previous cancer diagnosis Risk factors for lung cancer (e.g., smoking history, ethnicity, and asbestos exposure) Clinical tumor stage New primary cancer or recurrence Pathology accession number Principal clinician caring for the patient Other clinical information received
Macroscopic Operative procedure Specimen laterality Attached anatomical structures Accompanying specimens Block identification key Tumor site Tumor location Separate tumor nodules *Number of tumors* *Site* Maximum tumor dimension Macroscopic appearance of pleura overlying tumor Extent of direct spread of tumor to other tissues Distance of tumor to closest resection margin Tumor involves main bronchus within 20 mm of carina Lymph nodes *Site(s) and number of lymph nodes* Atelectasis/obstructive pneumonitis *Extent* Nonneoplastic lung Other relevant information and comments
Microscopic Histological tumor type *Adenocarcinoma classification* Histological grade Visceral pleural invasion *Extent of pleural involvement* Lymphovascular invasion *Vessel(s) involved* *Type of involvement* Perineural invasion
Pathological staging (AJCC seventh edition) Suffixes Primary tumor (T) Regional lymph nodes (N) Distant metastasis (M) Residual tumor status Completeness of surgical resection Diagnostic summary

Table 3.
Synoptic reporting of lung cancer.

clinical details and macroscopic, microscopic, and pathological staging as essential requirements. In addition, there should be an assessment of lymphovascular invasion and neurotropism and the presence of absence of satellite lesions; all these are shown in **Table 3**.

2. Management of lung cancer

2.1 Surgical management of primary lung cancer

Generally speaking, surgery is the best chance for stage I or II lung cancer patients [18]. Surgical oncology consultation is necessary for any patient being considered for local therapy. The general treatment plan, the essential imaging studies, and laboratory results should be determined before any nonemergency treatment is started. If patients cannot tolerate surgery or are inoperable, minimally invasive techniques, such as sublobar resection, can be a better choice [19]. Selected patients, including those who are not eligible for lobectomy and those with a peripheral nodule 2 cm or less with very low-risk features, are recommended to go through sublobar resection, either segmentectomy (preferred) or wedge resection. On the other hand, segmentectomy (preferred) or wedge resection should achieve parenchymal resection margins that are (1) 2 cm or more or (2) the size of the nodule or more.

2.2 Radiotherapy

The principles of radiation therapy in the NSCLC algorithm has been described thoroughly, including the following: general principles for early-stage, locally advanced, and advanced NSCLC; target volumes, prescription doses, and normal tissue dose constraints for early-stage, locally advanced, and advanced NSCLC; and RT simulation, planning, and delivery [20]. Treatment recommendations should be made by a multidisciplinary team. Because of the potential role of radiotherapy in all stages of NSCLC, whether it is a definitive treatment or palliative treatment is not known. Radiotherapy uses for NSCLC include, but are not limited to, (1) definitive treatment of locally advanced NSCLC, usually combined with chemotherapy; (2) definitive treatment of early NSCLC in patients with surgical contraindications; (3) partial preoperative or postoperative treatment of surgical patients; (4) treatment of limited recurrence and metastasis; and/or (5) palliative treatment of incurable NSCLC patients [21–23].

2.3 Immunotherapy and targeted therapy

Specific targeted therapies can be used to treat advanced NSCLC. Bevacizumab is a monoclonal antibody, targeting vascular endothelial growth factor, while ramucirumab is a recombinant monoclonal antibody that targets VEGF receptors. Cetuximab is a monoclonal antibody that targets EGFR. Erlotinib, gefitinib, and afatinib inhibit EGFR-sensitizing mutations; osimertinib inhibits both EGFR-sensitizing mutations and T790 M. ALK rearrangement, ROS1 rearrangement, and MET were all inhibited by crizotinib. Patients with ALK rearrangement are recommended to ceritinib which inhibits the IGF-1 receptor. Alectinib inhibits ALK and RET rearrangement. Brigatinib inhibits various ALK rearrangements and other targets. Dabrafenib/trametinib inhibits the BRAF V600E mutation; trametinib also inhibits MEK; both drugs inhibit different kinases in the RAS/RAF/MEK/ERK pathway [24, 25].

3. Role of PET-CT in lung cancer

3.1 Principles of PET-CT

PET-CT is a nuclear medicine technique that combines a positron emission tomography (PET) scanner with an X-ray computed tomography (CT) scanner. The anatomical imaging obtained by CT scan and the functional imaging obtained by PET (which depicts the spatial distribution of metabolic or biochemical activity in vivo) can achieve the same machine fusion more accurately, and the generated fusion image can be based on general software and control system to obtain 2D and 3D image reconstruction. Previously pure PET imaging cannot provide accurate anatomical positioning, and thus its value was limited, while PET-CT revolutionized medical diagnosis in many areas by increasing the accuracy of anatomical positioning in functional imaging. For example, the diagnosis and classification of benign and malignant tumors, the development of surgical plans, and the delineation of radiotherapy target areas have rapidly changed under the influence of PET-CT availability [26]. PET-CT-based grading staging has significantly changed clinical decisions; so many hospitals' nuclear medicine departments have gradually reduced the usage of traditional PET devices and replaced them with PET-CT. One of the barriers to the wider use of PET-CT is its relatively expensive price. Another obstacle is the difficulty and cost of producing and transporting of radiopharmaceuticals for PET imaging, which usually have a short half-life (e.g., radioactive fluorine-18). The half-life of (^{18}F) is used to track glucose metabolism (using fluorodeoxyglucose (FDG)) for only 106 minutes, and its production requires very expensive cyclotrons and radiopharmaceutical production lines [27].

3.2 Preoperative staging

Identifying the stage of lung cancer not only helps determine the appropriate treatment but also is essential for prognosis. Incorrect staging of lung cancer can lead to mistaken resections of benign nodules and early local or distant relapse after surgery with curative intent. Barbara randomly assigned patients referred for preoperative staging of NSCLC to either conventional staging plus PET-CT or conventional staging alone followed until death or for at least 12 months. They defined ineffective thoracotomy as any of the following: thoracotomy, pathologically confirmed mediastinal lymph node involvement (stage IIIA [N2]), stage IIIB or IV disease, or benign lung disease; exploratory thoracic incision; or thoracotomy in patients who have relapsed or died for any reason within 1 year after randomization. Ninety-eight patients were assigned to the PET-CT group and 91 to the conventional staging group. Sixty patients in the PET-CT group and 73 in the conventional staging group underwent thoracotomy ($P = 0.004$). Among these thoracotomies, 21 in the PET-CT group and 38 in the conventional staging group were futile ($P = 0.05$). Both groups had a reasonable thoracotomy and had similar survival. The use of PET-CT in the preoperative staging of NSCLC reduced the total number of thoracotomy and the number of ineffective thoracotomy, but did not affect overall mortality [28] (**Figure 2**).

3.3 Evaluation of treatment effect

Franco et al. conducted research aiming to evaluate the utility between PET-CT and the contrast-enhanced (CE) CT. The low-dose CT scans were performed for attenuation correction of the PET images, and the PET scanner was fully cross-calibrated, allowing accurate standard uptake value measurements. The protocols

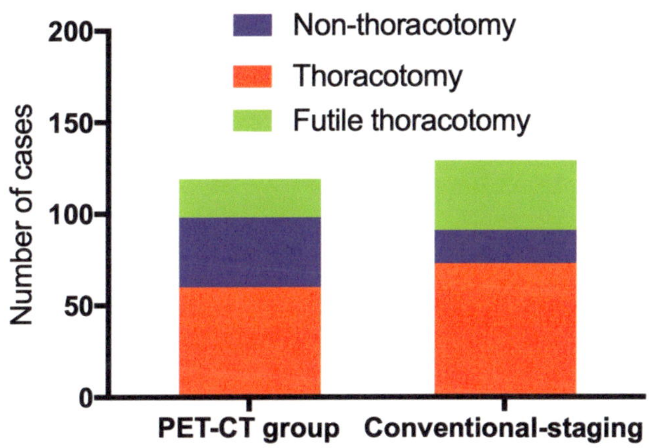

Figure 2.
Preoperative staging of NSCLC between PET-CT group and conventional staging group.

for CE-CT are the following: (1) all chest CT scans were performed according to the conventional low-dose chest multi-detection CT protocol, including head-to-tail orientation, arms raised on the head, single breath, and the amount of scan from the diaphragm level to the level directly above the chest entrance; and (2) the injected volume of contrast medium was tailored to the individual body weight: 60 mL at 2 mL/s for <50 kg or 80 mL at 2.5 mL/s at 50 kg or heavier with a fixed contrast delay of 35 seconds. The study enrolled 96 patients who received curative-intent treatment, and the results showed that the sensitivity, specificity, and positive predictive value for detecting cancer recurrence (95% confidence interval) were 0.88, 0.62, and 0.56 for PET-CT and 0.93, 0.72, and 0.64 for CE-CT, respectively, indicating that PET-CT is not superior to CE-CT in detecting cancer recurrence during 2 years after curative-intent treatment of non-small cell lung cancer [29].

3.4 Surveillance

Using systematic review and meta-analysis, Nie et al. evaluated the prognostic value of metabolic tumor volume (MTV) and total lesion glycolysis (TLG) for small cell lung cancer and used the pooled hazard ratio (HR) to measure the influence of MTV and TLG on survival. They found that patients with high MTV are associated with a significantly poorer prognosis OS and PFS, while high TLG is associated with a significantly poorer prognosis regarding OS for SCLC [30].

3.5 Guiding biopsy

When lung cancer is discovered, accurate staging at baseline is necessary to maximize patient benefit and cost-effective use of healthcare resources. Although CT remains a powerful tool for the staging of lung cancer, advances in combined imaging modalities, specifically PET-CT, have improved the baseline staging accuracy over that of CT alone [31]. FDG PET-CT has been considered a "metabolic biopsy" tool in the evaluation of nonlung lesions with indeterminate biopsy results [32]. PET-CT data coregistered with intraprocedural CT images could guide needle placement in the viable portion of the lesion and thus increase the chances of achieving a definitive diagnosis and CT-guided, fine-needle aspiration (FNA) biopsies performed with FDG PET scans of pulmonary lesions contributing substantially to the management and treatment of pulmonary disease [33].

4. PET-CT in lung cancer: teaching cases

4.1 Adenocarcinoma

Teaching point: adenocarcinoma mainly located in the peripheral segment and shows higher FDG uptake (**Figure 3**).

4.2 SCC

Teaching point: adenocarcinoma is mainly located in the central segment and shows moderate FDG uptake (**Figure 4**).

4.3 Large cell lung cancer

Teaching point: large cell lung cancer always shows moderate FDG uptake and diffused distribution (**Figure 5**).

4.4 Small cell lung cancer

Teaching point: small cell lung cancer shows a small mass with moderate FDG uptake (**Figure 6**).

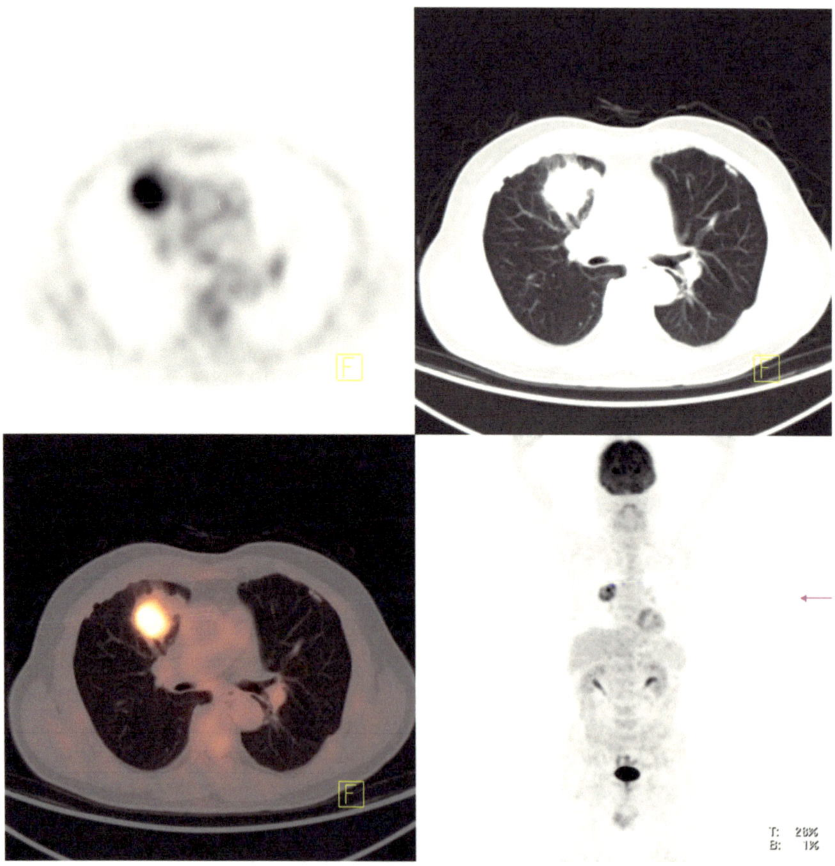

Figure 3.
Axial PET, CT, PET-CT, and MIP images in a patient of adenocarcinoma. An irregular mass showing higher FDG uptake in the lesion was discovered in the anterior segment of the right upper lobar.

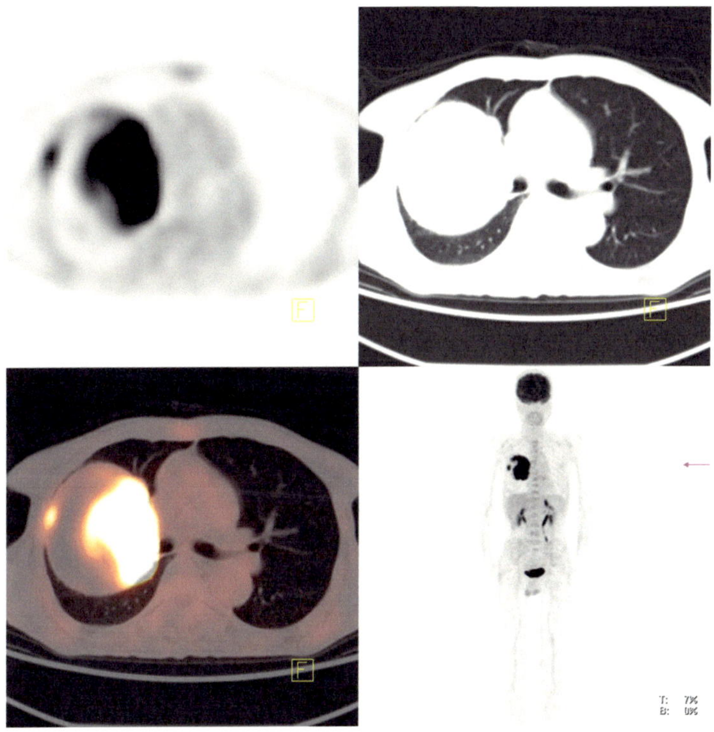

Figure 4.
Axial PET, CT, PET-CT, and MIP images in a patient of squamous cell carcinoma. An irregular mass showing moderate FDG uptake in the lesion was discovered in the central segment of the right lung, with inflammation around the malignant lung lesion.

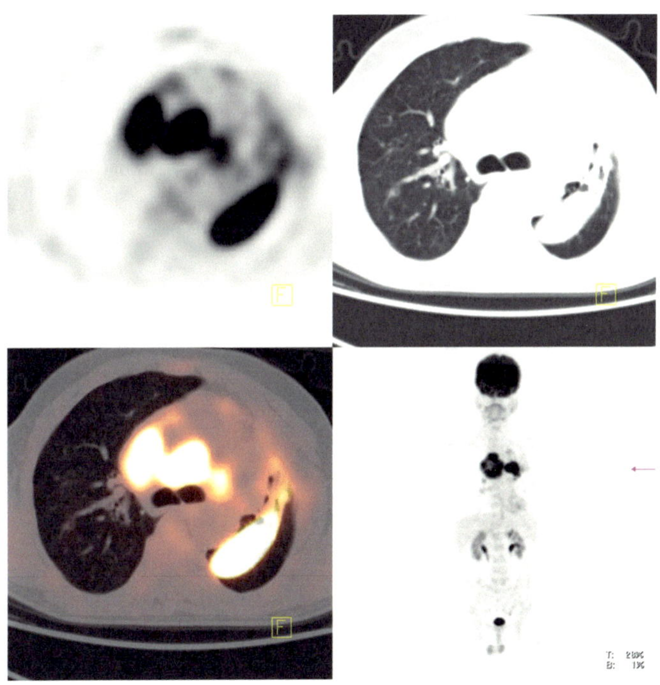

Figure 5.
Axial PET, CT, PET-CT, and MIP images in a patient of large cell cancer. Multisite masses showing higher FDG uptake in the lesion were discovered in the left and right lung field, with inflammation and enlarged lymph node in the mediastinum.

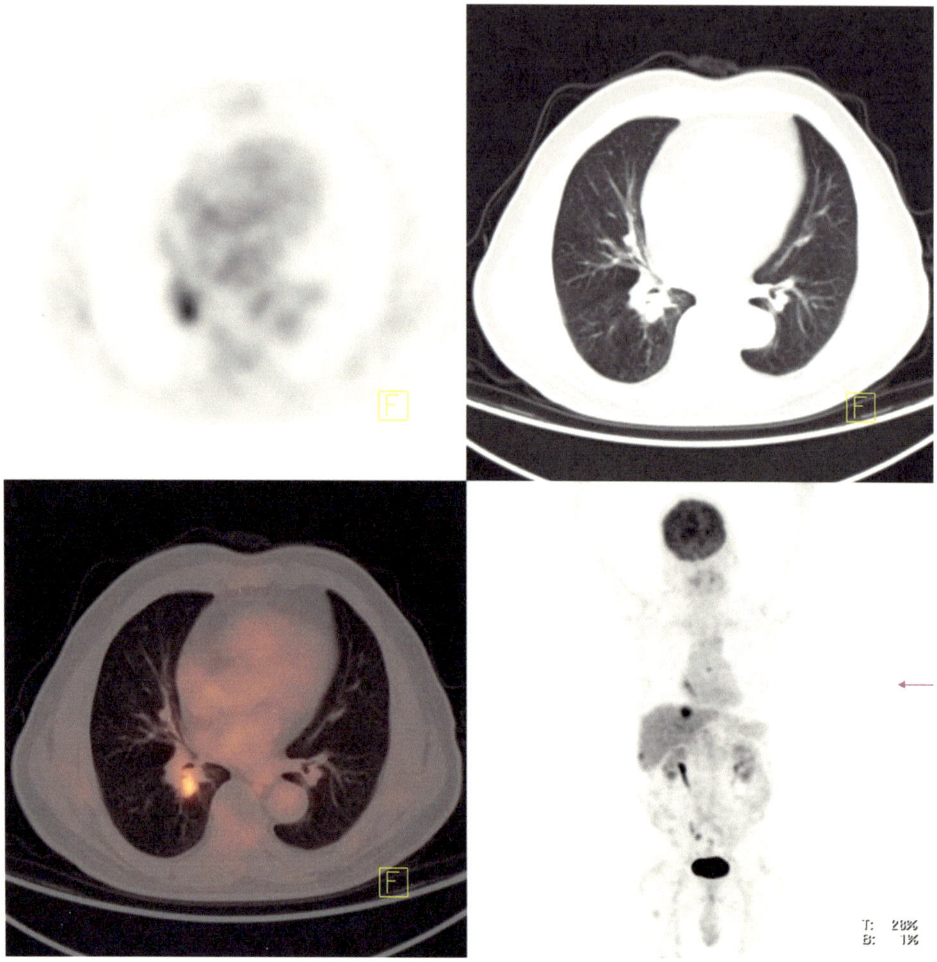

Figure 6.
Axial PET, CT, PET-CT, and MIP images in a patient of small cell lung cancer. Small mass located in the right hilar with slight FDG uptake in the lesion was discovered in the right lung field.

5. Conclusions

The current chapter focused on the PET-CT utility in lung cancer diagnosis and summarized the basic clinic utilities, including guiding to select the biopsy site, improving target delineation accuracy, evaluating disease progression on first-line therapy, and detecting hilar, mediastinal nodes and metastatic disease. PET-CT scans have been widely used to help evaluate the extent of disease and to provide more accurate staging and has been recommended by the NCCN. Patients with suspected malignant lung nodules should be scanned by PET-CT for accurate diagnosis of local or distant metastasis.

Acknowledgements

This work is supported by China Postdoctoral Science Foundation (No. 2019M653501), Initiation Foundation for Doctors of Yunnan Cancer Hospital (No. BSKY201706), Joint Special Fund from Yunnan Provincial Science and Technology Department-Kunming Medical University for Applied and Basic

Research (No. 2018FE001-150), the National Natural Science Foundation of China (No. 81960496) and the 100 Young and Middle-aged Academic and Technical Backbone Incubation Projects of Kunming Medical University.

Author details

Long Chen[1], Hua Sun[1] and Yunchao Huang[2]*

1 Department of PET/CT Center, Yunnan Cancer Hospital, The Third Affiliated Hospital of Kunming Medical University, Cancer Center of Yunnan Province, Xishan District, Kunming, Yunnan, People's Republic of China

2 Department of Thoracic Surgery I, Yunnan Cancer Hospital, The Third Affiliated Hospital of Kunming Medical University, Cancer Center of Yunnan Province, Xishan District, Kunming, Yunnan, People's Republic of China

*Address all correspondence to: huangyunch2017@126.com

References

[1] Bray F, Ferlay J, Soerjomataram I, Siegel RL, Torre LA, Jemal A. Global cancer statistics 2018: GLOBOCAN estimates of incidence and mortality worldwide for 36 cancers in 185 countries. CA: A Cancer Journal for Clinicians. 2018;**68**(6):394-424

[2] Siegel RL, Miller KD, Jemal A. Cancer statistics, 2018. CA: A Cancer Journal for Clinicians. 2018;**68**(1):7-30

[3] Johnson DH, Schiller JH, Bunn PA Jr. Recent clinical advances in lung cancer management. Journal of Clinical Oncology. 2014;**32**(10):973-982

[4] NCCN. 2019. Available from: https://www.nccn.org/professionals/physician_gls/pdf/nscl.pdf

[5] Seow WJ, Hu W, Vermeulen R, Hosgood Iii HD, Downward GS, Chapman RS, et al. Household air pollution and lung cancer in China: A review of studies in Xuanwei. Chinese Journal of Cancer. 2014;**33**(10):471-475

[6] Gibbs AR, Thunnissen FB. Histological typing of lung and pleural tumours: Third edition. Journal of Clinical Pathology. 2001;**54**(7):498-499

[7] Scagliotti GV, Parikh P, von Pawel J, Biesma B, Vansteenkiste J, Manegold C, et al. Phase III study comparing cisplatin plus gemcitabine with cisplatin plus pemetrexed in chemotherapy-naive patients with advanced-stage non-small-cell lung cancer. Journal of Clinical Oncology. 2008;**26**(21):3543-3551

[8] Johnson DH, Fehrenbacher L, Novotny WF, Herbst RS, Nemunaitis JJ, Jablons DM, et al. Randomized phase II trial comparing bevacizumab plus carboplatin and paclitaxel with carboplatin and paclitaxel alone in previously untreated locally advanced or metastatic non-small-cell lung cancer. Journal of Clinical Oncology. 2004;**22**(11):2184-2191

[9] Howlader NNA, Krapcho M, Miller D, Bishop K, Kosary CL, Yu M, et al. SEER Cancer Statistics Review, 1975-2014. National Cancer Institute; 2017

[10] Carter BW, Glisson BS, Truong MT, Erasmus JJ. Small cell lung carcinoma: Staging, imaging, and treatment considerations. Radiographics. 2014;**34**(6):1707-1721

[11] Brink I, Schumacher T, Mix M, Ruhland S, Stoelben E, Digel W, et al. Impact of [18F]FDG-PET on the primary staging of small-cell lung cancer. European Journal of Nuclear Medicine and Molecular Imaging. 2004;**31**(12):1614-1620

[12] Li C, Lu H. Adenosquamous carcinoma of the lung. OncoTargets and Therapy. 2018;**11**:4829-4835

[13] Noel-Savina E, Descourt R. Focus on treatment of lung carcinoid tumor. OncoTargets and Therapy. 2013;**6**:1533-1537

[14] Jiang M, Anderson T, Nwogu C, Tan D. Pulmonary malignant granular cell tumor. World Journal of Surgical Oncology. 2003;**1**(1):22

[15] Roesel C, Terjung S, Weinreich G, Hager T, Chalvatzoulis E, Metzenmacher M, et al. Sarcomatoid carcinoma of the lung: A rare histological subtype of non-small cell lung cancer with a poor prognosis even at earlier tumour stages. Interactive Cardiovascular and Thoracic Surgery. 2017;**24**(3):407-413

[16] Li T, Kung HJ, Mack PC, Gandara DR. Genotyping and genomic profiling of non-small-cell lung cancer: Implications for current and future therapies. Journal of Clinical Oncology. 2013;**31**(8):1039-1049

[17] Amin MB, Greene FL, Edge SB, Compton CC, Gershenwald JE, Brookland RK, et al. The Eighth Edition AJCC Cancer Staging Manual: Continuing to build a bridge from a population-based to a more "personalized" approach to cancer staging. CA: A Cancer Journal for Clinicians. 2017;**67**(2):93-99

[18] Howington JA, Blum MG, Chang AC, Balekian AA, Murthy SC. Treatment of stage I and II non-small cell lung cancer: Diagnosis and management of lung cancer, 3rd ed: American College of Chest Physicians evidence-based clinical practice guidelines. Chest. 2013;**143** (5 Suppl):e278S-e313S

[19] Brunelli A, Kim AW, Berger KI, Addrizzo-Harris DJ. Physiologic evaluation of the patient with lung cancer being considered for resectional surgery: Diagnosis and management of lung cancer, 3rd ed: American College of Chest Physicians evidence-based clinical practice guidelines. Chest. 2013;**143** (5 Suppl):e166S-e190S

[20] Lung Cancer Study Group. Effects of postoperative mediastinal radiation on completely resected stage II and stage III epidermoid cancer of the lung. The New England Journal of Medicine 1986;**315**(22):1377-1381

[21] Lutz ST, Jones J, Chow E. Role of radiation therapy in palliative care of the patient with cancer. Journal of Clinical Oncology. 2014;**32**(26):2913-2919

[22] Lutz ST, Lo SS, Chang EL, Galanopoulos N, Howell DD, Kim EY, et al. ACR Appropriateness Criteria(®) non-spine bone metastases. Journal of Palliative Medicine. 2012;**15**(5):521-526

[23] Gregoire V, Mackie TR. State of the art on dose prescription, reporting and recording in intensity-modulated radiation therapy (ICRU report No. 83). Cancer Radiothérapie. 2011;**15**(6-7):555-559

[24] Sandler AB, Johnson DH, Herbst RS. Anti-vascular endothelial growth factor monoclonals in non-small cell lung cancer. Clinical Cancer Research: An Official Journal of the American Association for Cancer Research. 2004;**10**(12 Pt 2):4258s-4262s

[25] Giaccone G. Epidermal growth factor receptor inhibitors in the treatment of non-small-cell lung cancer. Journal of Clinical Oncology. 2005;**23**(14):3235-3242

[26] Shao H, Ma X, Gao Y, Wang J, Wu J, Wang B, et al. Comparison of the diagnostic efficiency for local recurrence of rectal cancer using CT, MRI, PET and PET-CT: A systematic review protocol. Medicine (Baltimore). 2018;**97**(48):e12900

[27] Bertagna F, Albano D, Giovanella L, Giubbini R, Treglia G. F18-choline/C11-choline PET/CT thyroid incidentalomas. Endocrine. 2019;**64**(2):203-208

[28] Fischer B, Lassen U, Mortensen J, Larsen S, Loft A, Bertelsen A, et al. Preoperative staging of lung cancer with combined PET-CT. The New England Journal of Medicine. 2009;**361**(1):32-39

[29] Gambazzi F, Frey LD, Bruehlmeier M, Janthur WD, Graber SM, Heuberger J, et al. Comparing two imaging methods for follow-up of lung cancer treatment: A randomized pilot study. The Annals of Thoracic Surgery. 2019;**107**(2):430-435

[30] Nie K, Zhang YX, Nie W, Zhu L, Chen YN, Xiao YX, et al. Prognostic value of metabolic tumour volume and total lesion glycolysis measured by 18F-fluorodeoxyglucose positron emission tomography/computed tomography in small cell lung cancer: A systematic review and meta-analysis. Journal of Medical Imaging and Radiation Oncology. 2019;**63**(1):84-93

[31] Islam S, Walker RC. Advanced imaging (positron emission tomography

and magnetic resonance imaging) and image-guided biopsy in initial staging and monitoring of therapy of lung cancer. Cancer Journal. 2013;**19**(3):208-216

[32] Beggs AD, Hain SF, Curran KM, O'Doherty MJ. FDG-PET as a "metabolic biopsy" tool in non-lung lesions with indeterminate biopsy. European Journal of Nuclear Medicine and Molecular Imaging. 2002;**29**(4):542-546

[33] Collins BT, Lowe VJ, Dunphy FR. Initial evaluation of pulmonary abnormalities: CT-guided fine-needle aspiration biopsy and fluoride-18 fluorodeoxyglucose positron emission tomography correlation. Diagnostic Cytopathology. 2000;**22**(2):92-96

Section 3

Medical Imaging Processing Techniques

Chapter 5

Research in Medical Imaging Using Image Processing Techniques

Yousif Mohamed Y. Abdallah and Tariq Alqahtani

Abstract

Medical imaging is the procedure used to attain images of the body parts for medical uses in order to identify or study diseases. There are millions of imaging procedures done every week worldwide. Medical imaging is developing rapidly due to developments in image processing techniques including image recognition, analysis, and enhancement. Image processing increases the percentage and amount of detected tissues. This chapter presents the application of both simple and sophisticated image analysis techniques in the medical imaging field. This chapter also summarizes how to exemplify image interpretation challenges using different image processing algorithms such as k-means, ROI-based segmentation, and watershed techniques.

Keywords: medical, imaging, image processing technique

1. Introduction

Medical imaging is the process of producing visible images of inner structures of the body for scientific and medicinal study and treatment as well as a visible view of the function of interior tissues. This process pursues the disorder identification and management. This process creates data bank of regular structure and function of the organs to make it easy to recognize the anomalies. This process includes both organic and radiological imaging which used electromagnetic energies (X-rays and gamma), sonography, magnetic, scopes, and thermal and isotope imaging. There are many other technologies used to record information about the location and function of the body. Those techniques have many limitations compared to those modulates which produce images. Annually billions of images have been done globally for different diagnostic purposes. About half of them use ionizing and nonionizing radiation modulates [1]. Medical imaging produces the images of the internal structures of the body without invasive procedures. Those images were produced using fast processors and due to conversion of the energies arithmetically and logically to signals [2]. Those signals later are converted to digital images. Those signals represent the different types of tissues inside the body.

The digital images play a necessary role on a daily basis. The medical imaging processing refers to handling images by using the computer. This processing includes many types of techniques and operations such as image gaining, storage, presentation, and communication. The image is a function that signifies a measure of characteristics such as illumination or color a viewed sight. The digital images have several benefits such as faster and cheap processing cost, easy storing and communication, immediate quality assessment, multiple copying with reserving the quality, fast and cheap reproduction, and adaptable manipulation. The disadvantages of digital images are exploitation copyright, inability to resize with preserving the quality, the need of large-capacity memory, and the need of faster processor for manipulation [3].

An image processing technique is the usage of computer to manipulate the digital image. This technique has many benefits such as elasticity, adaptability, data storing, and communication. With the growth of different image resizing techniques, the images can be kept efficiently. This technique has many sets of rules to perform into the images synchronously. The 2D and 3D images can be processed in multiple dimensions. The image processing techniques were founded in the 1960s. Those techniques were used for different fields such as Space, clinical purposes, arts, and TV image improvement. In the 1970s with the development of computer system, the cost of image processing became less and faster. In the 2000s, the image processing became quicker, inexpensive, and simpler [4].

The human visual system is one of the most complex schemes that ever existed. This system allows living beings to organize and understand the many complex elements in their external environment. The visual system comprises of the eye that transmutes light into neural signals and the related parts of the brain that process those signals and excerpt essential data. The human eye is bilateral cylinder structures that are located anteriorly in the skull. The eyes are 2.5 cm in both crosswise and lengthwise diameters. In the middle of the eyeball, there is a blackened structure called the pupil. This system permits the light to cross the eye. This system narrows when exposed to a heavier light source. This reduces the light to the retina and enhances the visual process. There are many muscles surrounding the eye and that control the widening of the pupil. The eye always has some supporting structures called the sclera. The lens is a ligamentous part located behind the cornea. The

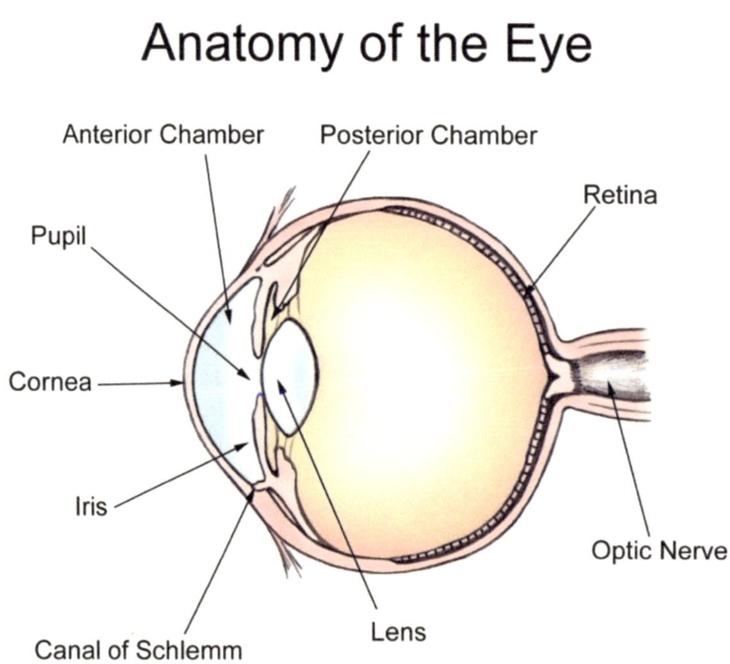

Figure 1.
The eyeball.

shape of the lens changes continuously due to muscle contraction [4, 5]. **Figure 1** shows the cross-sectional view of the eyeball.

The light concentrates into the middle part of the eye and focuses from the cornea and lens on retinae. The fovea emphases the image into the retina. Finally, the brain forms the details and colors using its perception through multiple processes.

2. Classification of digital images

The digital images have two main types of images. Raster image is described as a four-sided arrangement of frequently sampled values known as pixels. The digital images are usually inaccessible images and involve multifaceted color difference. The digital images have fixed resolution due to their pixels size. The digital images lose their quality in the resizing process due to some missing data. The digital images are used mainly in photography images because of their good color shades. The image-gaining instrument controls the resolution. The digital images include many formats such as BMP (Windows bitmap), TIFF (Tag Interleave Format), PCX (Paintbrush), PNG (Portable Network Graphics), etc. [6, 7].

A vector is described as a wrinkled and a bent object that is defined precisely by the computer. The vector has many qualities such as line width, dimension, and hue. The vectors are easily scalable images and can be reproduced in different magnitudes without change in its quality. The vectors are suitable for design, line painting, and diagrams.

3. Applications of digital image processing

The digital image processing has many applications in the medical field such as:

3.1 Medicine

In medicine, many techniques are used such as segmentation and texture analysis, which is used for cancer and other disorder identifications. Image registering and fusion methods are widely used nowadays specially in new modalities such as PET-CT and PET-MRI. In the field of bioinformatics, telemedicine and the formatless compression techniques are used to communicate the image remotely [1–5].

3.2 Forensics

The common techniques used in this field are edge detection, pattern matching, denoising, security, and biometric purposes such as identity, face, and fingerprint documentation. Forensics is based on the database information about the individuals. Forensics matches the input data (fingerprint, eye, photo, etc.) with the database to define the person identity [2].

4. Medical imaging systems

Medical imaging systems use the signals received from the patient to produce images. Medical imaging systems use both ionizing and nonionizing sources.

4.1 X-ray imaging systems

Since the discovery of X-rays by the German scientist Roentgen, X-rays have been used to image the body parts for diagnostic purposes. In X-ray tube, the electrons are produced in cathode through a thermal emission process and are accelerated through a potential difference of 50–150 KV. The electrons hit the anode to produce the X-rays. Only 1% of this energy is converted to X-rays, and the remaining amount is changed to heat (**Figure 2**) [3].

In the X-ray machines, the images are produced in 2D plans of the examined part of the body. The fluoroscopy system is used to scan the moving organs. The acquired images can be displayed, stored, and communicated through different machines. Computed radiography (CT) uses image receptor to produce the image. X-rays accompany a screen covered with a storage phosphor device. The mammography imaging is used to differentiate between the breast tissues and different diseases. Mammography imaging uses lower energy compared with bony structure imaging. The range of potential difference used is 15–40 kV (**Figure 3**) [2–16].

4.2 Computed tomography (CT)

In this modality, the images are produced in multiple dimensions rather than the conventional radiography. CT scanner produces multiple slices of the body tissues in different directions. In CT scanner, the patient is placed inside its aperture and scanned by a rotating X-ray tube in all directions (**Figure 4**) [6].

4.3 Nuclear medicine

This imaging modality uses the radioisotopes to produce images about the functions of the different structures such as the heart, kidney, and liver. The radioisotopes are labeled by pharmaceutical materials to be guided to the certain organs. The patient's emitted photons are received in the detectors and convert into signals. Those signals are converted to interpretable digital images. There are many types of nuclear medicine scanning modalities such as planar, tomographic, and positron emissions. The planar emission produces 2D images. Both of the tomographic and the positron emissions produce 3D images (**Figure 5**) [5].

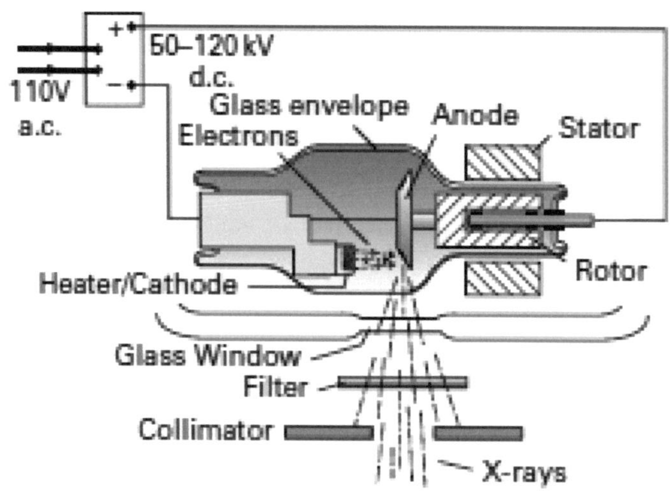

Figure 2.
X-rays tube.

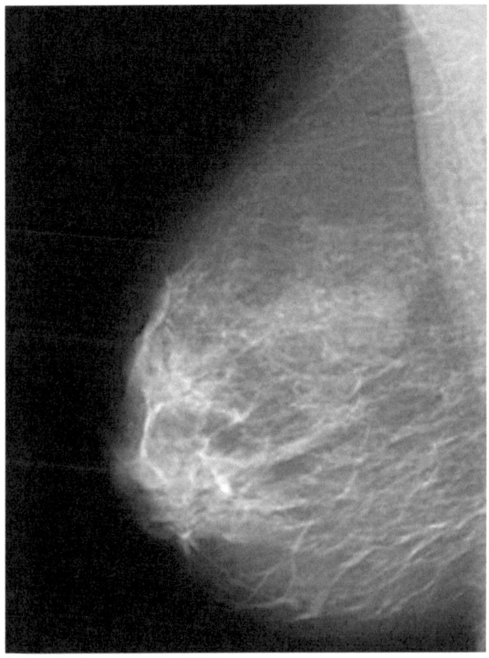

Figure 3.
Mammography image.

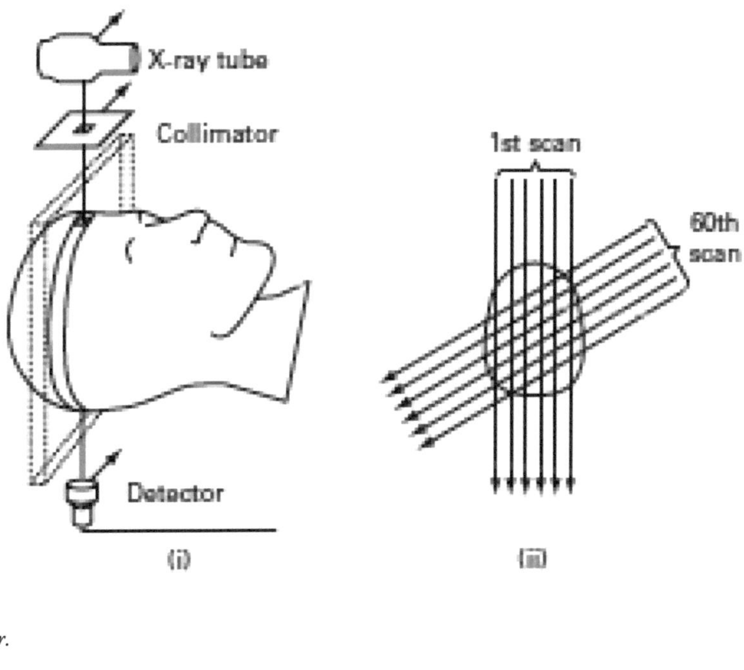

Figure 4.
CT scanner.

4.4 Ultrasound

Ultrasound is a technique, which uses high-frequency sound waves to produce images of the internal structure of the body from the returned echoes. Ultrasound is similar to the location determination technique, which is used by some animals like bats and whales in the nature. Ultrasound is transmitted in high-frequency pulses into the body using a transducer as those waves travel through the body tissues.

Some of those waves are absorbed and some reflect back. The reflected waves are received by the transducer and converted into electric signals. Those electric signals are converted into digital ones and pass through the computer system. The computer system uses the arithmetic and logic calculation to form the 2D image of the scanned structures. In the ultrasonic system, thousands of pulses are sent per each millisecond. There are many imaging techniques used to enhance the ultrasound images (**Figure 6**) [1–6].

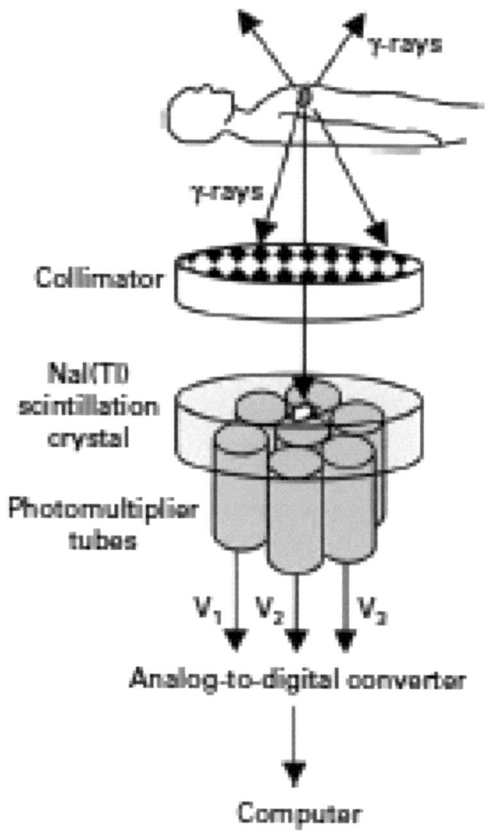

Figure 5.
Nuclear medicine imaging.

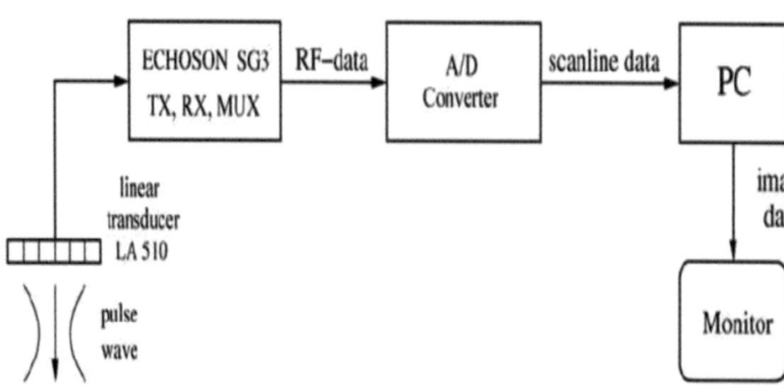

Figure 6.
Ultrasound imaging diagram.

5. Fundamentals of digital image processing

The images are classified according to different qualities such as illumination, contrast, entropy, and signal-to-noise ratio. The histogram is the simplest image processing technique. The image display does not change the image quality. The grayscale histogram considers the basic type of the images that are used to evaluate and to improve the images. The histogram is a scheme showing the pixels' values and not their locations. The gray-level histogram shows whether an image is generally shady or bright (**Figure 5**). The mean pixel value is obtained from the histogram by summing the produced pixel values and consistent bin altitude and dividing by the entire number of pixels [7, 8]. Histogram equalization is used to compare many images acquired on definite bases. The technique works by changing the histogram to become smooth, identical, and balanced (**Figure 7**).

The mean value of central pixel intensity is designated to the ideal brightness. Any intensity above or below makes the image darker or brighter. Signal-to-noise ratio (SNR) of an image is used to associate the level of the anticipated signal to the level of the contextual signal. Signal-to-noise ratio (SNR) is defined as the ratio of signal intensity to noise intensity. Signal-to-noise ratio (SNR) calculates from the image in an up-front method. The mean intensity of the image is expressed as the square of the mean of the pixel value (Eq. (1)).

$$SNR = \frac{P_{signal}}{P_{noise}} \tag{1}$$

where p is the average power.

5.1 Image enhancement

Image enhancement is a technique used to improve the image quality and perceptibility by using computer-aided software. This technique includes both objective and subjective enhancements. This technique includes points and local operations. The local operations depend on the district input pixel values. Image enhancement has two types: spatial and transform domain techniques. The spatial techniques work directly on the pixel level, while the transform technique works on Fourier and later on the spatial technique (see **Figures 8** and **9**) [9].

5.2 Image segmentation

Image segmentation is a technique of segregating the image into many parts. The basic aim of this segregation is to make the images easy to analyze and interpret

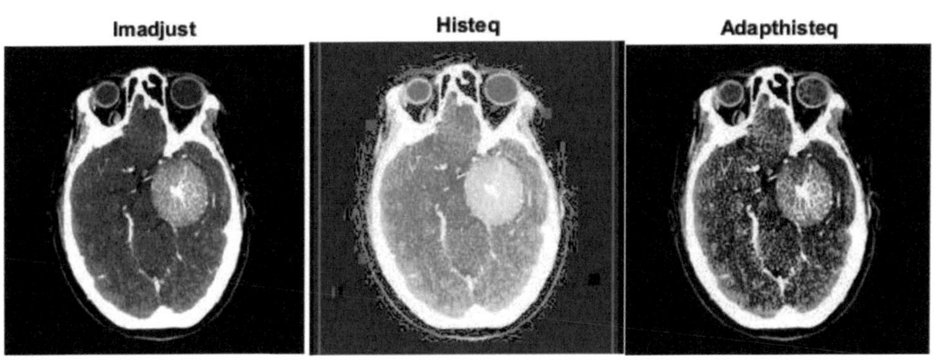

Figure 7.
Sagittal MRI image of a head had enhanced using (i) image adjustment, (ii) histogram equalization, and (iii) adaptive histogram equalization [8].

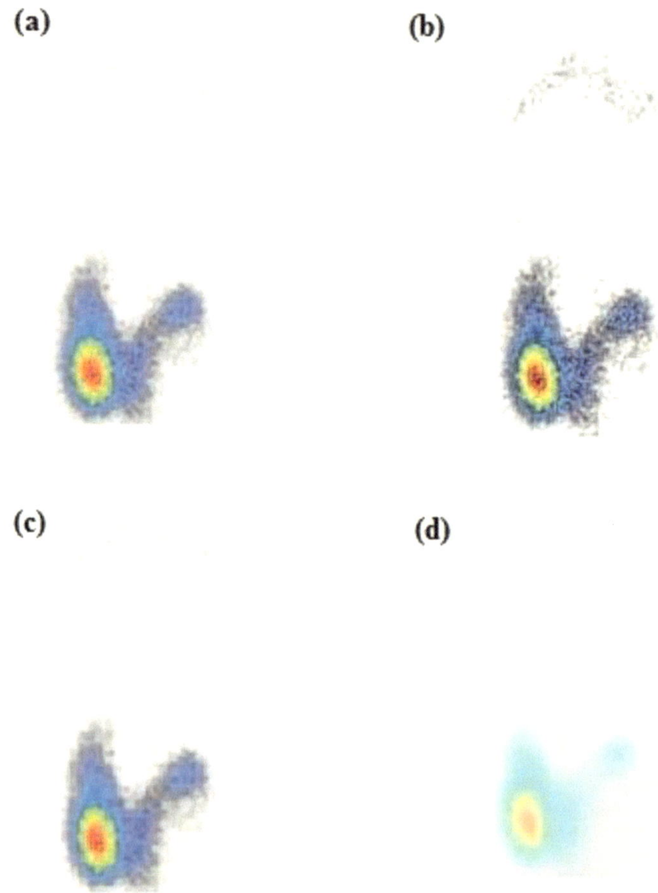

Figure 8.
Edge-aware local contrast manipulation of thyroid scan images (a), (b) edge threshold, (c) original image and (d) reduced contrast −0.5 [12].

with preserving the quality. This technique is also used to trace the objects' borders within the images. This technique labels the pixels according to their intensity and characteristics. Those parts represent the entire original image and acquire its characteristics such as intensity and similarity. The image segmentation technique is used to create 3D contour of the body for clinical purposes. Segmentation is used in machine perception, malignant disease analysis, tissue volumes, anatomical and functional analyses, 3D-rendered technique, virtual reality visualization and anomaly analysis, and object definition and detection (**Figure 10**) [12–14].

Image segmentation is divided into kinds: (i) local segmentation and (ii) global segmentation. The local segmentation works particularly in one subdivision of the image. This technique has a fewer number of pixels compared to the global type. The global segmentation works in the whole image as one unit. This technique has more pixels to manipulate. Segmentation can be divided into methods:

1. region method;

2. boundary method; and

3. Edge method [14].

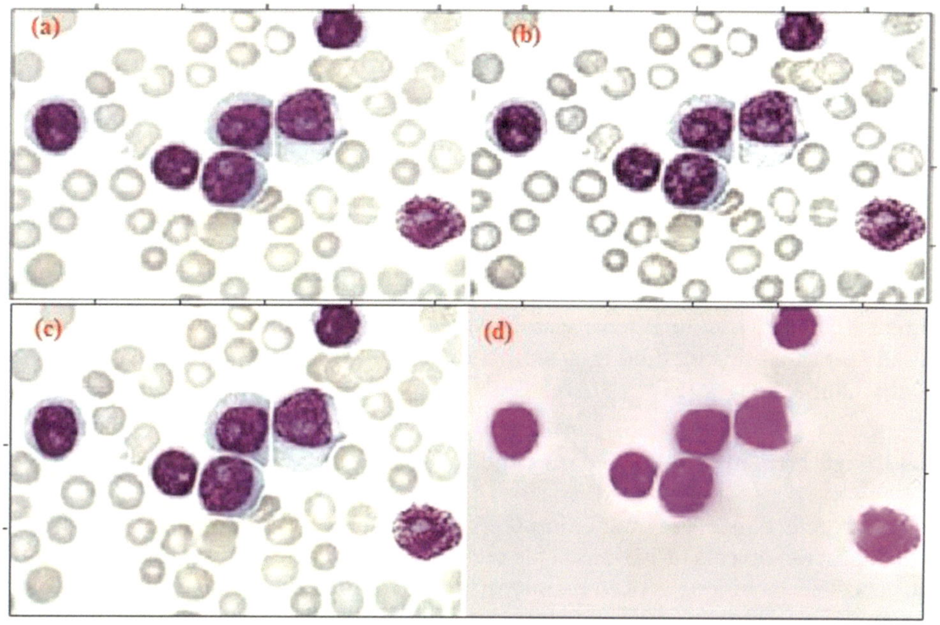

Figure 9.
Edge-aware local contrast manipulation of leukemia cell images (a) and (c) original image, (b) Edge threshold, and (d) Reduced contrast −0.5 [13].

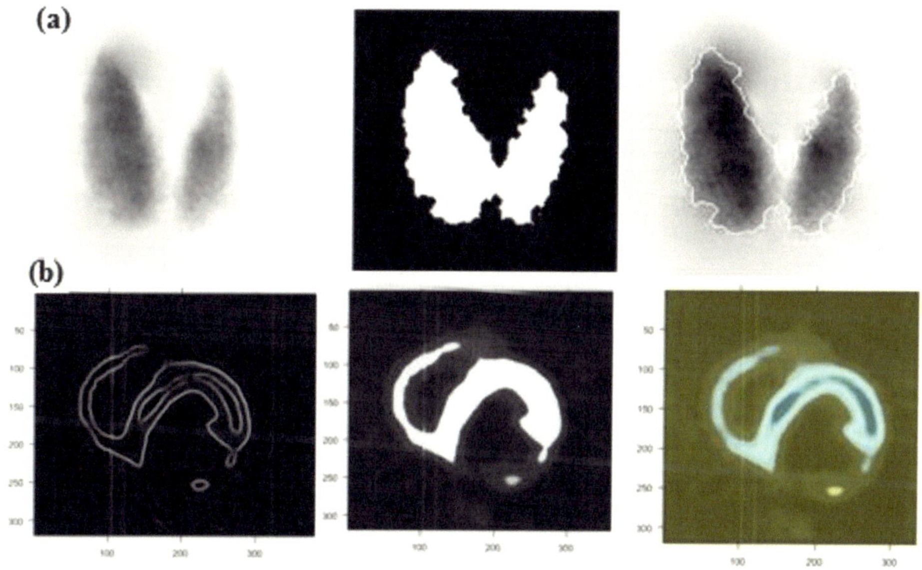

Figure 10.
Segmentation process of (a) thyroid gland and heart [3].

5.3 Image segmentation based on thresholding

Thresholding segmentation depends on the threshold value to convert the gray color-based image into black and white [4]. There are many other techniques applied in radiology in order to rebuild or reslice the images such as Otsu's and k-means techniques [5, 6]. Threshold method is useful for establishing the borders of solid objects in a dark background. Threshold techniques need presence of differences between the object's and background's intensities. There are three types of thresholding methods. Those methods include global, adaptive, and histogram-built selection threshold. The global threshold is broader and used for all segmentation techniques. The global threshold (θ) calculates using binarization procedure as in the following equation (Eq. (2)):

$$f(x) = \begin{cases} 1\, if\, f\ (m,n) \geq \theta \\ 0 \end{cases} \tag{2}$$

The adaptive or fixed threshold segments image faster if the region of interest contains unique intensity and is different from the background. The disadvantage of this method is its simplicity and inability to process the multichannel images [15].

5.4 Image segmentation based on edge detection

Edge detection is a segmentation technique that uses border recognition of strictly linked objects or regions. This technique identifies the discontinuity of the objects. This technique is used mainly in image study and to recognize the parts of image where a huge variation in intensity arises.

5.5 Some types of edge detection

5.5.1 Roberts kernel

Roberts kernel is a technique used for determining the difference between two close pixels. Precisely it is called forward differences. This technique can find the edges in high noised images; it is calculated using first-order fractional derivative and cross-gradient operator (Eqs. (3) and (4)) (**Figure 11**) [21].

$$\frac{\partial f}{\partial x} = f\ (i,j) - f\ (i+1,j+1) \tag{3}$$

$$\frac{\partial f}{\partial x} = f\ (i+1,j) - f\ (\mathrm{i},j+1) \tag{4}$$

The fractional derivative can be applied into two 2 × 2 matrices. In this situation, Roberts masks are calculated as in Eq. (5):

$$G_x = \begin{bmatrix} -1 & 0 \\ 0 & 1 \end{bmatrix} \text{ and } G_y = \begin{bmatrix} 0 & -1 \\ 1 & 0 \end{bmatrix} \tag{5}$$

5.5.2 Prewitt kernel

This technique is based on the idea of central difference. This technique is better than Roberts operator (**Figure 11**). Assume that matric has arrangement of pixels [i, j] as in Eq. (6):

$$\begin{bmatrix} a_0 & a_1 & a_2 \\ a_7 & [i,j] & a_3 \\ a_6 & a_5 & a_4 \end{bmatrix} \tag{6}$$

The fractional derivative of Prewitt operator is computed as in Eq. (7):

$$G_x = (a_2 + ca_3 + a_4) - (a_0 + ca_7 + a_6) \tag{7}$$

where c is constant and expresses the pixels closed to the center of the image. G_x and G_y are the calculations at [i, j]. When c equals 1, the Prewitt operator is calculated as in **Figure 10** and Eq. (8) [15, 16]:

$$G_x = \begin{bmatrix} -1 & -1 & -1 \\ 0 & 0 & 0 \\ 1 & 1 & 1 \end{bmatrix} \text{ and } G_y = \begin{bmatrix} -1 & 0 & 1 \\ -1 & 0 & 1 \\ -1 & 0 & 1 \end{bmatrix} \tag{8}$$

5.5.3 Sobel kernel

This technique can be dependent on the central difference which tends toward the central pixels in average. This technique can be expressed as 3 × 3 matric to the first derivative of Gaussian kernel. This technique is calculated as shown in Eqs. (9)–(12) [20–22]:

$$G_x = (a_2 + 2a_3 + a_4) - (a_0 + 2a_7 + a_6) \tag{9}$$

and

$$G_y = (a_6 + 2a_5 + a_4) - (a_0 + 2a_1 + a_2) \tag{10}$$

The Sobel masks are the following:

$$G_x = \begin{bmatrix} -1 & -2 & -1 \\ 0 & 0 & 0 \\ 1 & 1 & 1 \end{bmatrix} \text{ and } G_y = \begin{bmatrix} -1 & 0 & 1 \\ -2 & 0 & 2 \\ -1 & 0 & 1 \end{bmatrix} \tag{11}$$

The Sobel is better than Prewitt in noise reduction [18]. This technique is used in the functional imaging modality such as nuclear medicine. In the study of red blood cell images, the unraveling of strictly neighboring cells is considered difficult issues due to the background noise. This affects the interpreting processes and makes them difficult to diagnose by the physician. Segmentation can solve such problems and identify those red cells easily (see **Figure 12**) [17].

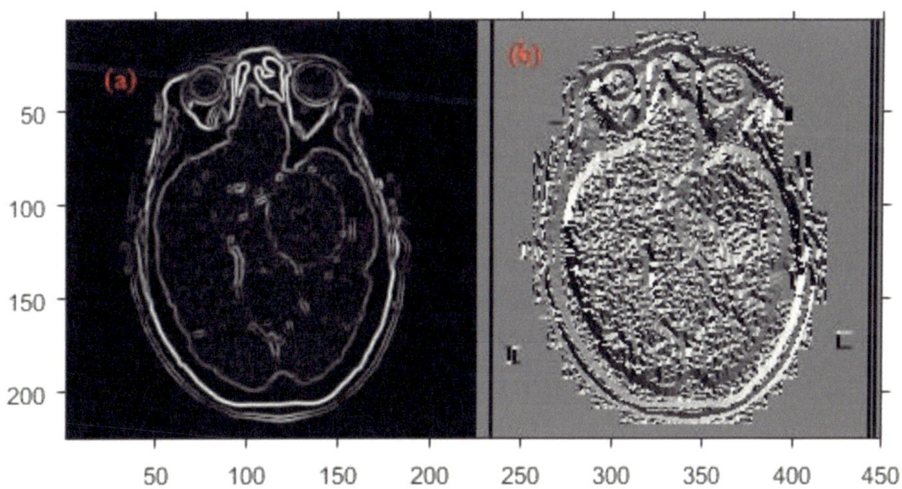

Figure 11.
Prewitt edge detection technique, (a) gradient magnitude, and (b) gradient direction.

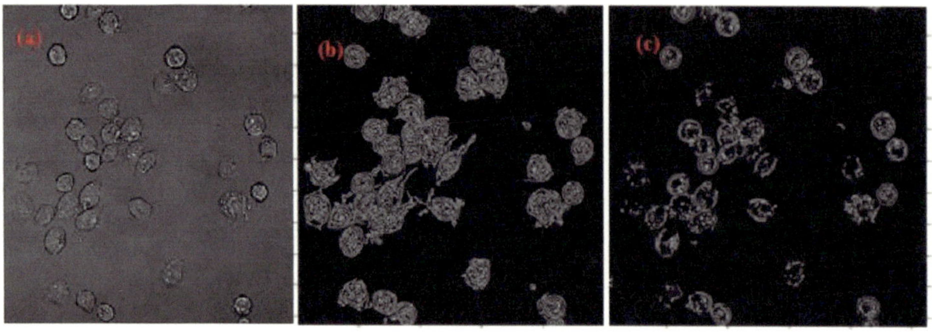

Figure 12.
Red blood cell segmentation using edge detection: (a) original image and (b) Sobel and (c) Prewitt techniques.

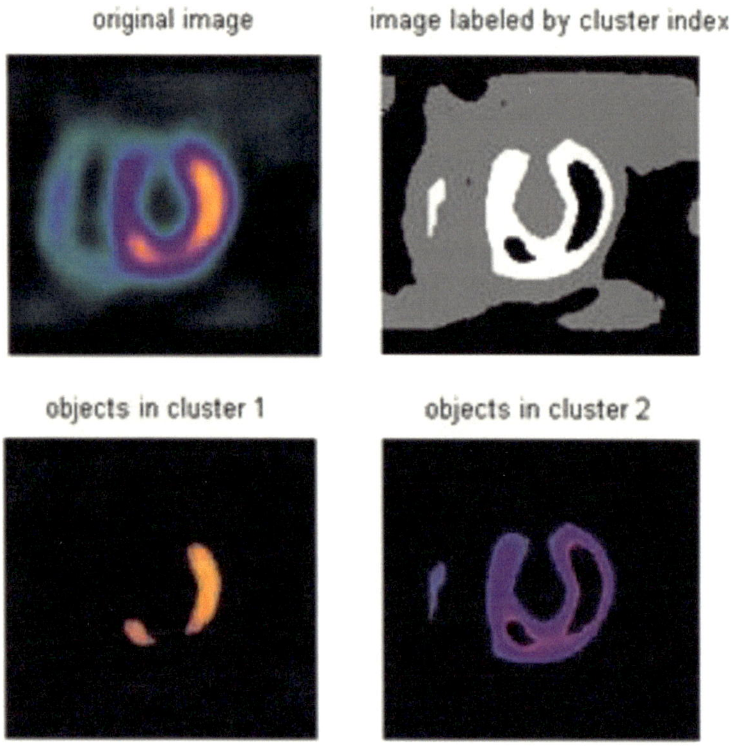

Figure 13.
k-means segmentation technique of nuclear medicine images.

5.6 k-means segmentation

k-means cluster is a technique of vector and signal valuations. This technique subdivides the image into n parts and into k clusters in which each observation fits to a cluster with a similar mean. k-means clustering tends to find clusters of comparable spatial extent. Given a set of comments (x1, x2, ..., xn), where each comment is a d-dimensional actual vector, k-means clustering aims to subdivide the n observations into k ($\leq$ n) sets S = {S1, S2, ..., Sk} so as to minimize the within-cluster sum of squares (Eqs. (12) and (13)) [16].

$$\arg min_S \sum_{i=1}^{k} \sum_{x \in S_i} \|x-\mu_i\|^2 = \arg min_S \sum_{i=1}^{k} |S_i VarS_i \quad (12)$$

where $\boldsymbol{\mu}_i$ is the mean of points in S_i.

$$\arg min_S \sum_{i-1}^{k} \frac{1}{2|S_i|} \sum_{x1y \in S_i} \|x - y\|^2 \quad (13)$$

k-means technique can be applied in large databases because of its simplicity. This technique is used in economical, stargazing, cultivation, and computer perception (**Figure 13**) [17–19].

6. Conclusion

Images are the method of expression of the data in pictographic form. Images consist of various small elements called pixels. Each pixel has a specific position and value. Geometric image signifies an image arithmetically with geometrical primitives such as lines. Each image is saved in a specific file format, which consists of two parts, the heading and the data. Imaging processing techniques is a group of approaches that are used for handling the images by computer. The objective of segmentation is the partition of the images into important portions. Local segmentation deals with the partition of the images into small parts within the images. Global segmentation deals with the assembly of those partitions. Image segmentation works in three methods, which are region, border, and edge. Region method is used to examine images and region class of neighboring pixels. Thresholding segmentation uses the histogram and threshold value of pixels. Image edge techniques are used to analyze the images at borders or discontinuing. Those techniques include Roberts, Prewitt, Sobel, and Frei-Chen.

Acknowledgements

The authors are thankful to the Deanship of Scientific Research, at Majmaah University, for funding this research.

Conflict of interest

There are no conflicts of interest.

Author details

Yousif Mohamed Y. Abdallah[1]* and Tariq Alqahtani[2]

1 Radiological Science and Medical Imaging Department, College of Applied Medical Science, Majmaah University, Majmaah, Saudi Arabia

2 Medical Equipments Technology Department, College of Applied Medical Science, Majmaah University, Majmaah, Saudi Arabia

*Address all correspondence to: y.yousif@mu.edu.sa

References

[1] Abdallah Y. Improvement of sonographic appearance using HAT-TOP methods. International Journal of Science and Research (IJSR). 2015;**4**(2):2425-2430. DOI: http://dx.doi.org/10.14738/jbemi.55.5283

[2] Abdallah Y. Increasing of edges recognition in cardiac scintigraphy for ischemic patients. Journal of Biomedical Engineering and Medical Imaging. 2016;**2**(6):40-48. DOI: http://dx.doi.org/10.14738/jbemi.26.1697

[3] Abdallah Y. Application of Analysis Approach in Noise Estimation, Using Image Processing Program. Germany: Lambert Publishing Press GmbH & Co. KG; 2011. pp. 123-125

[4] Abdallah Y, Yousef R. Augmentation of X-rays images using pixel intensity values adjustments. International Journal of Science and Research (IJSR). 2015;**4**(2):2425-2430

[5] Abdallah Y. Increasing of Edges Recognition in Cardiac Scintography for Ischemic Patients. Germany: Lambert Publishing Press GmbH & Co. KG; 2011. pp. 123-125

[6] Abdallah YM. History of medical imaging. Archives of Medicine and Health Sciences. 2017;**5**:275-278. DOI: 10.4103/amhs.amhs_97_17

[7] Abdallah Y. An Introduction to PACS in Radiology Service: Theory and Practice. Germany: LAP LAMBERT Academic Publishing; 2012. ISBN: 978-3846588987

[8] Abdallah Y. Application of Analysis Approach in Noise Estimation: Using Image Processing Program. LAP LAMBERT Academic Publishing; 2011. ISBN: 978-3847331544

[9] Abdallah Y. Computed Verification of Light and Radiation Field Size Superimposition On Cobalt-60 machine, Verification of Fields Size using Image Processing Technique. Germany: LAMBERT Academic Publishing GmbH & Co. KG; 2010. ISBN: 9783838399096

[10] Abdallah Y, Mohamed E. Improvement of bone scintography image using image texture analysis. Frontiers in Biomedical Sciences. 2016;**1**(1):1-6

[11] Abdallah Y. Segmentation of salivary glands in nuclear medicine images using edge detection tools. Journal of Biomedical Engineering and Medical Imaging. 2016;**3**(2):1-6. DOI: http://dx.doi.org/10.14738/jbemi.32.1702

[12] Abdallah Y, Mohamed S. Automatic recognition of leukemia cells using texture analysis algorithm. International Journal of Advanced Research (IJAR). 2016;**4**(1):1242-1248

[13] Abdallah Y, Algaddal A, Alkhir M. Enrichment of ultrasound images using contrast enhancement techniques. International Journal of Science and Research (IJSR). 2015;**4**(1):2381-2385

[14] Abdallah Y. Increasing the precision of edges recognition in static renal scintography. Indian Journal of Applied Research (IJAR). 2015;**4**(7):270-273

[15] Abdallah Y, Wagiallah E, Yousef M. Improvement of nuclear cardiology images for ischemic patients using image processing techniques. SMU Medical Journal. 2015;**2**(2):1-9

[16] Abdallah Y. Lungs detection in ventilation and perfusion scintigraphy using watershed transform. International Journal of Electronics Communication and Computer Engineering (IJECCE). 2015;**2**(3):416-419